# The Emerging Global Health Crisis

## Noncommunicable Diseases in Low- and Middle-Income Countries

COUNCIL *on*
FOREIGN
RELATIONS

Independent Task Force Report No. 72

Mitchell E. Daniels Jr. and
Thomas E. Donilon, *Chairs*
Thomas J. Bollyky, *Project Director*

# The Emerging Global Health Crisis
Noncommunicable Diseases
in Low- and Middle-Income Countries

# Task Force Members

Task Force members are asked to join a consensus signifying that they endorse "the general policy thrust and judgments reached by the group, though not necessarily every finding and recommendation." They participate in the Task Force in their individual, not institutional, capacities.

David B. Agus
*University of Southern California*

J. Brian Atwood
*Humphrey School of Public Affairs*

Samuel R. Berger
*Albright Stonebridge Group*

Karan Bhatia
*General Electric Company*

Thomas J. Bollyky
*Council on Foreign Relations*

Nancy G. Brinker
*Susan G. Komen*

Binta Niambi Brown
*Harvard Kennedy School*

Barbara Byrne
*Barclays*

Jean-Paul Chretien
*U.S. Navy*

Mitchell E. Daniels Jr.
*Purdue University*

Steve Davis
*PATH*

Thomas E. Donilon
*O'Melveny & Myers*

Ezekiel J. Emanuel
*University of Pennsylvania*

Daniel R. Glickman*
*Aspen Institute*

Eric P. Goosby
*University of California, San Francisco*

Vanessa Kerry*
*Seed Global Health*

Michael J. Klag
*Johns Hopkins Bloomberg School of Public Health*

*The individual has endorsed the report and signed an additional view.

Risa Lavizzo-Mourey
*Robert Wood Johnson Foundation*

Christopher J.L. Murray
*University of Washington*

Elizabeth G. Nabel
*Brigham and Women's Hospital*

David Satcher
*Morehouse School of Medicine*

Donna E. Shalala
*University of Miami*

Ira S. Shapiro
*Ira Shapiro Global Strategies LLC*

Tommy G. Thompson
*Thompson Family Holdings*

# Contents

# Foreword

The attention of the world is currently fixed on three countries in West Africa, and understandably so. Emerging infectious diseases such as Ebola pose a serious threat not just to the societies and the men, women, and children in the immediate vicinity of an outbreak, but to countless others around the world owing to globalization.

At the same time, it remains the case that the gravest health threats facing low- and middle-income countries are less the obscure viruses or ancient plagues that dominate the news cycle and international relief efforts so much as diseases we understand and could address but too often fail to combat.

Once thought to be challenges for affluent countries alone, cardiovascular diseases, cancer, diabetes, and other noncommunicable diseases (NCDs) are now the leading cause of death and disability in developing countries. In 2013, these diseases killed eight million people before their sixtieth birthdays in these countries. The chronic nature of NCDs means patients may be sick for many years and require extensive medical care. The economic costs, in terms of both immediate health-care costs and lost productivity, are high and rising in low- and middle-income countries, threatening their continued development and prosperity.

Possibly because NCDs constitute a gathering rather than a dramatic or imminent crisis, the international response has been woefully inadequate. The United States has no dedicated programs or budget for addressing NCDs globally. Despite the efforts of the World Health Organization and the United Nations to elevate the priority of these diseases, aid for NCDs represented just 1.2 percent of total development assistance for global health in 2011. The urgency of this situation led the Council on Foreign Relations (CFR) to convene an Independent Task Force on Noncommunicable Diseases—its first ever devoted to a global health matter.

The report begins by examining NCDs in developing countries and the factors driving their increasing prevalence. The analysis reveals that NCDs are rising faster, affecting younger populations, and having worse health and economic outcomes than seen in developed countries. This growing epidemic, the report says, is not merely the unfortunate byproduct of higher incomes and declining infectious disease rates. The report credits the confluence of several dramatic trends for driving the increase in NCDs: unprecedented rates of urbanization, global integration of consumer markets, and advances in longevity in still-poor countries that lack sufficient health systems to adjust.

The report also assesses the case for increased U.S. focus on NCDs. That assessment includes an examination of the countries that receive significant U.S. health assistance and finds that premature burden of death and disability in many of these countries is heavily NCD-related. The Task Force concludes that deeper U.S. involvement on NCDs is needed to ensure the continued effectiveness and credibility of U.S. global health programs in these countries, to advance U.S. trade with emerging economies, and to build institutional capacity in states of U.S. strategic concern.

There is much the United States can do to help developing countries meet the NCD challenge at relatively modest cost. U.S. efforts should focus on the specific NCDs and risk factors that are especially prevalent among the working-age poor in developing countries and for which there are existing low-cost interventions that can leverage current U.S. global health programs. Based on those criteria, the Task Force offers short-, medium-, and long-term recommendations for action. These range from prevention of cardiovascular disease to helping countries establish effective tobacco controls.

The report concludes with a call for the United States to take two immediate steps. First, the Task Force urges the U.S. government to undertake a serious examination of its global health programs and consider expanding their mandate. Second, the Task Force recommends that the United States convene other leading actors and potential partners on addressing NCDs —national governments, international institutions, philanthropic foundations, nongovernmental organizations, and private companies—to develop a well-prioritized and sustainable plan for collective action on NCDs in low- and middle-income countries.

I would like to thank the Task Force's chairs, Mitchell E. Daniels Jr. and Thomas E. Donilon, for their dedication to and active involvement in this important project. I am thankful to all of the Task Force members and observers whose diverse expertise in global health, trade, economic development, and foreign policy helped shape this report.

My thanks also extend to Chris Tuttle, CFR's Task Force Program director, and his predecessor Anya Schmemann for their guidance and tireless support for this project since its inception. Finally, I would like to extend my thanks to Project Director Thomas J. Bollyky for his dedicated work in producing this valuable report on this critical issue.

**Richard N. Haass**
*President*
Council on Foreign Relations
December 2014

# Acknowledgments

The report of the Independent Task Force on Noncommunicable Diseases (NCDs) is the product of a great deal of effort by the members, observers, and supporters of the Task Force, and I am grateful for the time, attention, and expertise that each of these individuals devoted to this project.

In particular, I would like to thank our distinguished co-chairs, Mitchell E. Daniels Jr. and Thomas E. Donilon, for their leadership. Mitch and Tom have deep experience and expertise in the conduct and priorities of U.S. policy, but neither comes from a specialized global health background. Instead, they came to this project with open minds, a healthy skepticism about new U.S. commitments, and an insistence on data-driven and scrupulously rigorous analysis. That analytical approach enhanced the quality of this report and helped produce the unanimous consensus for the strong recommendations included therein. It has been a pleasure to work with these co-chairs and their teams.

I am also grateful for the Task Force members' and observers' invaluable guidance. Many members took the time to provide detailed comments and feedback throughout the Task Force process and the report has been much improved for their efforts.

I acknowledge in particular the help and support that I received in producing this report from Christopher J.L. Murray, a Task Force member and the director of the Institute for Health Metrics and Evaluation (IHME) at the University of Washington, and his very able colleagues, Joseph Dieleman and Tara Templin. The data on NCDs and their associated health risks that underlies much of the analysis in this report originates from the groundbreaking Global Burden of Disease project that Chris leads at IHME. The analysis, figures, and projections included in the report are nearly all original and the product of many long hours from Joe and Tara and their patient collaboration with me. I am deeply indebted to them.

I much appreciate the detailed comments I received from David Fidler at Indiana University Mauer School of Law and Ruth Levine at the Hewlett Foundation, whom I asked informally to serve as external reviewers of this report. David and Ruth are two of the smartest, most practical-minded people working in global health and their insights on this report were further evidence of those qualities. I am also grateful to Joshua Michaud, associate director for global health at the Kaiser Family Foundation, for his assistance sifting through the 2013 U.S. global health aid budget. I am thankful to Ursula Bauer and Donald Shriber of the U.S. Centers for Disease Control and Prevention, who met with and briefed the Task Force at the outset of this project.

I also received help and support from CFR members. The CFR National and Corporate Programs organized consultations in Washington, DC, and in four cities on the West Coast to solicit CFR members' views and suggestions on the Task Force and its report. My thanks to Task Force members David B. Agus and Chris Murray for participating in the events in Los Angeles and Seattle, respectively.

I am grateful to many at CFR. The Publications team assisted in editing the report and readied it for publication. The Communications, Corporate, and Outreach teams all worked to ensure that the report reaches the widest audience possible. Additionally, CFR's Meetings and Events teams in both New York and Washington deserve thanks for ably coordinating launch events for the report.

I was blessed with excellent CFR staff support throughout this Task Force. I am particularly thankful to Caroline Andridge and Jerusha Murugen, my research associates during this project, for their customarily tireless and excellent work. Veronica Chiu, Daniel Chardell, Marisa Shannon, and Kristin Lewis from CFR's Independent Task Force Program were extremely helpful and ensured the Task Force ran smoothly, from organizing meetings to editing drafts. I also thank the interns that worked on this project for their enthusiasm and valuable contributions: Justin Jin, Alison Pease, and Scott Weathers.

I am particularly appreciative of Task Force Program Director Christopher M. Tuttle for his invaluable guidance and support throughout this project. Chris is truly a joy to work with. I also thank his predecessor, Anya Schmemann, who helped get this project off to a strong start.

I am grateful to CFR President Richard N. Haass for giving me the opportunity to direct this effort. With most donors' priorities elsewhere, few in the foreign policy community have taken on NCDs in any sustained way. Richard deserves much credit for his willingness to have CFR lead on this long-neglected and important issue.

Finally, I thank Bloomberg Philanthropies for its generous support of this Task Force and Kelly Henning for her active engagement throughout the project.

**Thomas J. Bollyky**
*Project Director*

# Acronyms

| | |
|---|---|
| ACE | angiotensin-converting-enzyme |
| DAH | development assistance for health |
| DALY | disability-adjusted life year |
| FCTC | Framework Convention on Tobacco Control |
| FDA | Food and Drug Administration |
| FY | fiscal year |
| GAVI | Global Alliance for Vaccines and Immunization |
| GBD | Global Burden of Disease |
| GDP | gross domestic product |
| GHI | U.S. Global Health Initiative |
| GTSS | Global Tobacco Surveillance System |
| HBV | hepatitis B virus |
| HIV/AIDS | human immunodeficiency virus infection and acquired immune deficiency syndrome |
| HPV | human papillomavirus |
| IHME | Institute for Health Metrics and Evaluation |
| IMF | International Monetary Fund |
| MNCH | maternal, newborn, and child health |
| NCD | noncommunicable disease |
| NCI | National Cancer Institute |
| NHLBI | National Heart, Lung, and Blood Institute |
| NIH | National Institutes of Health |
| PAHO | Pan American Health Organization |
| PEPFAR | President's Emergency Plan for AIDS Relief |

| | |
|---|---|
| **R&D** | research and development |
| **TB** | tuberculosis |
| **UN** | United Nations |
| **UNICEF** | United Nations Children's Fund |
| **USAID** | United States Agency for International Development |
| **WHO** | World Health Organization |

*Task Force Report*

# Executive Summary

The biggest global health crisis in low- and middle-income countries is not the one you might think. It is not the exotic parasites, bacterial blights, or obscure tropical viruses that have long occupied international health initiatives and media attention. It is cancer, cardiovascular disease, diabetes, and other noncommunicable diseases (NCDs), which killed more than eight million people before their sixtieth birthdays in low- and middle-income countries in 2013 alone. Unless urgent action is taken, the NCD crisis emerging in developing countries will worsen and become harder to address with each passing year.

The rise of NCDs in low- and middle-income countries is not merely the byproduct of success—increasing incomes, reductions in infectious diseases such as HIV/AIDS, or greater adoption of unhealthy western lifestyles. Recent improvements in life expectancy explain why more people in developing countries get NCDs. They do not, however, explain why so many people in these countries are developing NCDs so much younger and with such worse outcomes than in wealthier nations. Rates of obesity, consumption of fatty foods, and physical inactivity are rising in low- and middle-income countries, but they remain much lower than in most high-income countries. Premature death and disability from NCDs are increasingly associated with poverty in emerging nations, just as they are in wealthier countries.

The factors fueling the emergence of NCDs are the combination of dramatic changes in urbanization, global trade and consumer markets, and longevity that occurred over decades in wealthy nations but are happening much faster in still-poor countries. These changes are outpacing the ability of developing-country governments to establish the health and regulatory systems necessary to adjust. With these trends expected to persist or accelerate, the toll of NCDs on working-age populations will increase in these countries (Figure 1).

*FIGURE 1: PREMATURE (UNDER AGE SIXTY) DEATHS FROM NCDS*

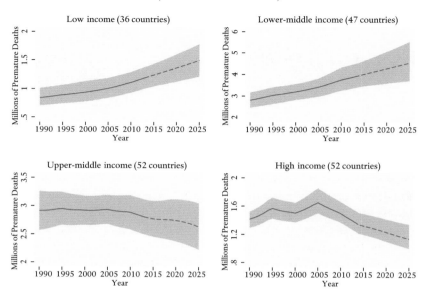

*Underlying Data Source:* Institute for Health Metrics and Evaluation, Global Burden of Disease Study 2013.[1]

U.S. interests will be affected by the rise of NCDs in low- and middle-income countries because of their human, economic, and strategic consequences. More patients will get sick, suffer longer, require more medical care, and die young. Given the scale of these trends, the results will reverberate. At the household level, it will mean less income, catastrophic health expenditures, and potential impoverishment. At the national level, it will mean lower productivity and competitiveness, higher health and welfare expenditures, and a potential missed opportunity for the demographic dividend that lifted the fortunes of many higher-income countries. At the global level, the World Economic Forum projects that the NCD epidemic will inflict $21.3 trillion in losses in developing countries over the next two decades—a cost nearly equal to the total aggregate economic output ($24.5 trillion) of these countries in 2013. These economic consequences will undercut potential U.S. trade partners and allies, and may reduce domestic support for foreign governments of strategic interest to the United States.

This outcome is not inevitable. Despite much higher rates of obesity and physical inactivity, premature death and disability from NCDs have declined dramatically in the United States and other high-income countries. The difference? Mostly cheap and effective prevention, management, and treatment tools and policies that are not widely implemented in developing countries, but could be by using well-established global health strategies. Yet the international community has struggled to act.

The urgency of this situation has led the Council on Foreign Relations (CFR) to convene an Independent Task Force on Noncommunicable Diseases in Low- and Middle-Income Countries—its first ever devoted to a global health matter. The charge of this Task Force is to assess the case for greater U.S. engagement on the NCD crisis in developing countries and recommend a practical and scalable strategy for intervention.

The last time that the world confronted a global health challenge that caused such a large number of premature adult deaths and so disproportionately affected low- and middle-income countries was HIV/AIDS. The United States led the global response to that disease, and the world rallied to its side. The U.S. government launched the President's Emergency Plan for AIDS Relief (PEPFAR) and worked with other donors and partners to establish the Global Fund to Fight AIDS, Tuberculosis, and Malaria. These programs have delivered treatment to millions, saved many lives, and inspired a dramatic increase in international support for addressing other global health challenges from malaria to family planning to maternal and child health. It is an accomplishment of which every American may feel deeply proud.

This Task Force finds that leadership on the new emerging global health crisis of NCDs in low- and middle-income countries is vital to U.S. interests—in improved global health, increased trade and development, and U.S. standing in the world. The means by which that leadership is demonstrated, however, must be different from U.S. interventions on HIV/AIDS.

The United States cannot solve the NCD crisis emerging in developing countries. Determining health priorities and allocating resources in the face of this crisis are decisions for national governments. Yet, working with like-minded partners, the United States can slow the rise of this epidemic, lessen its worst effects, and help provide national governments with the time and technical assistance needed to tackle this emerging crisis sustainably on their own.

Figure 2 depicts two projections. The first (red line) is the expected increase in premature (defined in this report as under age sixty) deaths from NCDs in the forty-nine countries where the United States

FIGURE 2: PROJECTED PREMATURE NCD DEATHS IN FORTY-NINE
U.S. PRIORITY COUNTRIES, 2014–2025

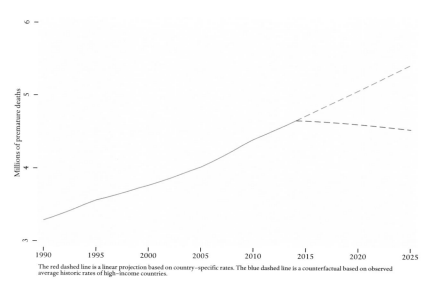

The red dashed line is a linear projection based on country–specific rates. The blue dashed line is a counterfactual based on observed
average historic rates of high–income countries.

*Underlying Data Source:* Institute for Health Metrics and Evaluation, Global Burden of Disease Study 2013.

currently has significant global health investments. The second (blue
line) is the decrease in premature mortality that would occur if those
countries improved NCD prevention and treatment at the same rate
that the average high-income country did between 2000 and 2013. The
difference between those projections is 5,166,984 lives over the next
eleven years. If this outcome could be achieved or even approached, the
results would be comparable to other successful U.S.-supported initiatives on childhood immunization and HIV.[2]

The Task Force recommends that U.S. investments in NCDs focus
initially on the specific diseases and risk factors that are (a) especially
prevalent among the working-age poor in developing countries and for
which (b) effective and low-cost interventions exist that are (c) amenable to collective action and (d) can leverage existing U.S. global health
programs and platforms. The Task Force applied these criteria to the
NCDs that are causing large numbers of premature deaths in low- and
middle-income countries but far fewer in high-income countries. That
assessment provides the basis for our recommendations in three areas.

- *Challenges on which U.S. leadership would make a tremendous difference now*: primary and secondary prevention of cardiovascular disease; tobacco control; hepatitis B vaccination to prevent liver cancer; and human papillomavirus (HPV) vaccination and screening programs to prevent cervical cancer
- *Challenges on which U.S. leadership would make a tremendous difference soon*: frugal diagnostic and curative care strategies for treatable and curable cancers such as leukemia and breast cancer; and better diabetes management for low-resource settings
- *Shared challenges on which U.S. collaboration with developing countries and the private sector could help*: population-based strategies to reduce poor diets and nutrition, physical inactivity, and obesity; integration of mental health into primary care; and low-cost chronic care programs and technologies

The recommendation to increase U.S. engagement on NCDs is not one to which this Task Force comes lightly. The United States already does much to address global health, and its resources are not infinite. Yet given strong U.S. interests in addressing the rising NCD epidemic in developing countries and the availability of proven, cost-effective interventions, our conclusion is unavoidable. The time to act is now.

This report proceeds as follows. Sections one and two examine the emerging crisis of NCDs in developing countries and the factors behind its rise. Section three assesses U.S. interests in increased engagement on NCDs internationally. Section four presents a practical, data-driven set of recommendations for that engagement. Each recommendation is accompanied by a case for U.S. investment.

The report concludes with two immediate steps that the United States should take. First, the U.S. government should undertake a serious examination of its global health priorities and spending and act to ensure their continued effectiveness in advancing U.S. interests. In the forty-nine countries with the most U.S. global health investment, the U.S. government spent $44.17 in aid for each year of life lost to disability and early death from HIV/AIDS in 2010 (as measured in disability-adjusted life years, or DALYs), $4.21 per DALY lost to malaria, and $1.82 per DALY lost to tuberculosis, but only $0.02 per DALY lost to NCDs. If the United States devoted the same resources it spends at the lower end of this range—$236 million on tuberculosis in fiscal year (FY) 2014—to NCDs, it would go a long way toward implementing the recommendations outlined in this report. The United States should consider the potential for additional funds to respond to the changing needs of these countries and the feasibility of building on the positive legacy of PEPFAR-funded programs by expanding their mandate from disease-focused goals to more outcome-oriented measures for improving health.

The costs and the burden of action on NCDs should not be borne by the United States alone. The second step that the United States should take is to convene the leading actors and potential partners for addressing NCDs—national governments, intergovernmental and international institutions, philanthropic foundations, nongovernmental organizations (NGOs), and private companies, especially large-scale employers operating in heavily affected countries. The purpose of this convening should be to develop a practical, well-prioritized, and sustainable plan for collective action on the global health crisis of NCDs in low- and middle-income countries.

# The Rising Epidemic of NCDs
# in Low- and Middle-Income Countries

When most people in developed countries think of the world's biggest health challenges, they envision a small child in a dusty, rural village suffering from an exotic parasite or bacterial blight. But increasingly, that image is wrong. Instead, it is the working-age woman living in an urban slum in a low- or middle-income country suffering from cervical cancer, or the father of young children dying of a stroke—noncommunicable diseases that were once thought to confront wealthy nations alone.[3]

NCDs are rising fast in low- and middle-income countries (Figure 3). As defined by the World Health Organization (WHO), NCDs are a broad category of chronic diseases and conditions that cannot themselves be

*FIGURE 3: DEATHS CAUSED BY NCDS IN LOW- AND MIDDLE-INCOME COUNTRIES*

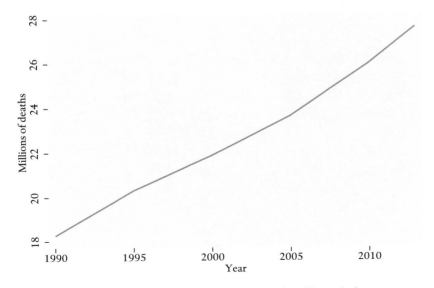

*Data Source:* Institute for Health Metrics and Evaluation, Global Burden of Disease Study 2013.

spread from person to person, although they may be caused by viruses or bacteria that can. In developing countries, four NCDs dominate. Cardiovascular diseases, cancer, and chronic respiratory illnesses cause 80 percent of the deaths and two-thirds of the disability from NCDs in these countries (Figure 4). Rates of diabetes are increasing the fastest, particularly in Central America, Africa, the Middle East, and Oceania.

Cancer, diabetes, stroke, and these other NCDs long ago became a challenge for developed countries as well, but the epidemiological transition happening in developing countries differs in speed, scale, and consequence. The rise of NCDs in these countries is not simply a result of reductions in the plagues and parasites that kill children and adolescents.[4] Death and disability from NCDs in low- and lower-middle-income countries is increasing faster than the rate of decline from communicable diseases. The trajectories of many NCDs depend on the wealth of the country where one lives. The death and disability wrought by heart disease, stroke, breast cancer, and other NCDs (measured in Table 1 as disability-adjusted life years, or DALYs) are subsiding in developed countries but increasing fast in developing countries.

*FIGURE 4: CAUSE OF NCD DEATHS IN LOW- AND MIDDLE-INCOME COUNTRIES*

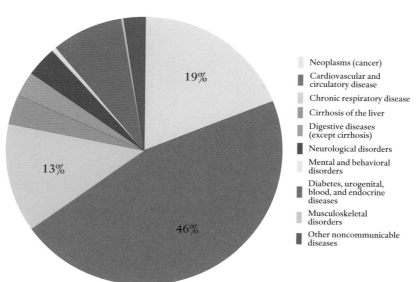

*Data Source:* Institute for Health Metrics and Evaluation, Global Burden of Disease Study 2013.

*TABLE 1: PERCENTAGE CHANGE IN DALYS: 1990–2010*

| | Low income | Lower-middle income | Upper-middle income | High income |
|---|---|---|---|---|
| All communicable diseases | -14% | -27% | -47% | -23% |
| All NCDs | 42% | 38% | 18% | 9% |
| Ischemic heart disease | 71% | 61% | 42% | -21% |
| Cerebrovascular disease | 45% | 43% | 16% | -17% |
| Lung cancer | 78% | 56% | 52% | 7% |
| Breast cancer | 124% | 58% | 55% | 1% |
| Cervical cancer | 28% | 19% | 18% | -16% |
| Leukemia | 54% | 30% | -7% | 1% |

*Data Source:* Institute for Health Metrics and Evaluation, Global Burden of Disease Study 2010.

NCDs are also arising faster in younger populations in low- and middle-income countries than in wealthy states. Most of the death and disability from NCDs in emerging countries (as depicted in Figure 5, in DALYs) occurs in working-age people (those under the age of sixty). In many low-income countries, particularly in Africa, that proportion rises to 80 percent or higher.

NCDs are not only rising faster and in younger populations in low- and middle-income countries, they are also yielding worse outcomes (Figure 6). NCDs that are preventable or treatable in developed countries are often death sentences in developing countries. Whereas cervical cancer can largely be prevented in developed countries thanks to the HPV vaccine, in sub-Saharan Africa and South Asia it is the leading cause of death from cancer among women;[5] likewise, 90 percent of children with leukemia in high-income countries can be cured, but 90 percent of those with that disease in the world's twenty-five poorest countries die from it.[6] Nine out of ten chronic obstructive respiratory deaths worldwide occur in low- and middle-income countries.[7]

The differences in developed- and developing-country survival rates are particularly high for cancers that have good prognoses with early diagnosis, as well as coronary heart disease and diabetes, for which high-income-country patients have access to relatively cheap and effective treatments.[8] Angiotensin-converting-enzyme (ACE) inhibitors, beta-blockers, and insulin are long off-patent, but still unavailable or inaccessible in low- and middle-income countries due to high costs and limited supply.[9] Overall, the WHO estimates that developing countries account for 90 percent of the nine million premature deaths from NCDs.[10]

The frequent onset of NCDs among young people and the bad health outcomes that result are having devastating economic and social consequences in low- and middle-income countries. The chronic nature of most of these diseases means patients are sick and

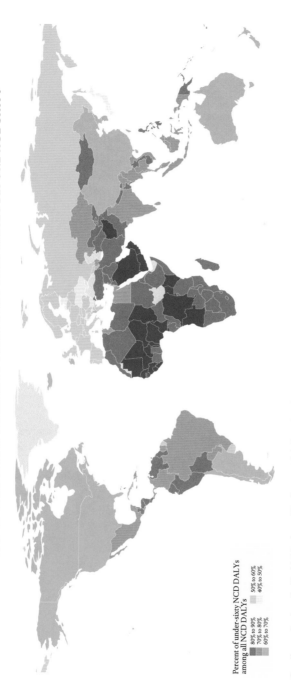

FIGURE 5: PROPORTION OF DEATH AND DISABILITY FROM NCDS THAT ARISES BEFORE AGE SIXTY

Percent of under-sixty NCD DALYs
among all NCD DALYs

80% to 90%          50% to 60%
70% to 80%          40% to 50%
60% to 70%

Data Source: Institute for Health Metrics and Evaluation, Global Burden of Disease Study 2010.

FIGURE 6: AGE-STANDARDIZED NCD DEATH RATES IN ADULTS

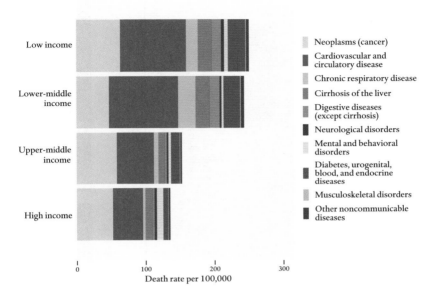

Data Source: Institute for Health Metrics and Evaluation, Global Burden of Disease Study 2013.

suffer longer and also seek and require more medical care and hospitalization. The effects are felt at the household, national, and global levels (Exhibit 1).

On a household level, NCDs consume budgets through out-of-pocket health-care costs as well as absenteeism and foregone income for patients and caregivers.[11] In Sudan, households with diabetic children devote 65 percent of household expenditures to their care.[12] In rural Ghana, minimum-wage earners with diabetes spend 60 percent of their incomes on insulin.[13] To cover these costs, households take unsecured loans, deplete savings, or sell assets, all of which put families on precarious financial footing. The rates of catastrophic health expenditures in India for households with a male family member suffering from cancer or cardiovascular disease are 44 percent and 24 percent, respectively.[14] Premature death and disability from NCDs robs families of their primary wage earners.

Many diseases experienced by mothers can spread to children; NCDs, despite their designation as noncommunicable, are proving

*EXHIBIT 1: EFFECTS OF NCDS IN LOW- AND MIDDLE-INCOME COUNTRIES*

## Individuals and Households

- Premature death and disability
- Lost household income, potential impoverishment
- Health expenditures, including catastrophic
- Loss of savings and assets
- Greater likelihood of children developing NCDs

## Health Systems

- Poor health outcomes
- Diminished capacity to address other health needs
- Resources to retool health systems to chronic, preventative care
- Health labor force and training demands
- Increased demand for high-cost medical interventions

## National Economies and Governments

- Reduced labor supply
- Lower productivity and competitiveness
- Lower tax revenues
- Increased health and social welfare expenditures
- Lost demographic dividend
- Eroded institutional capacity
- Political pressure from unmet population needs

*GLOBAL AND REGIONAL EFFECTS*

## Poorer Global Health

## Reduced International Trade and Development

## Potential for Political Instability

no different.[15] Diabetes and hypertension can impair fetal growth and development, and increasing evidence shows a mother's physiological condition during pregnancy predisposes her newborns to adult diseases such as coronary heart disease and stroke.[16]

On a national level, early onset of chronic illnesses consumes scarce health-care resources and undermines the capacity of developing-country health systems to respond to infectious and nutritional diseases and other health threats.[17] This is particularly true in the poorest countries in sub-Saharan Africa and South Asia, where malnutrition, HIV/AIDS, and other communicable diseases remain significant problems.[18]

The rise of NCDs, if unaddressed, can breed political instability and dissatisfaction with governments. The national health systems in most low- and middle-income countries are not equipped to meet the demand for primary and chronic care of NCDs. This retooling will require disease surveillance and registries; community-based health promotion and prevention programs; better health-care financing; more nurses, primary care physicians, and specialists; diagnostic laboratories; and cost-effective medical technologies and health-care delivery models. As the NCD epidemic accelerates and the health and economic outcomes worsen, popular demands for this health system retooling will increase, particularly among the middle class. In 2013, mass protests rocked Brazil; demonstrators railed against an underfunded, overcrowded health system and its chronic shortages of beds, medicines, and doctors.[19]

Government health and welfare expenditures are not the only NCD-related economic costs for countries. Premature death and disability from NCDs saps low- and middle-income countries' labor supply and diminishes workforce productivity.[20] This makes it harder to capitalize on the demographic dividend that would otherwise occur from reduced child mortality, better family planning, and having a larger proportion of young, working-age people relative to developed countries (Figure 7). As a result, the wealth generation and productive investments that would arise from that dividend are reduced or lost. Consumer spending and savings, especially among the rising middle class, suffers. Increased health expenditures and lower productivity diminish national competitiveness and foreign direct investment.[21] Tax revenues decline.

Given the scale of the emerging NCD epidemic in low- and middle-income countries, the effects of these diseases on individuals and households, health systems, and national economies and governments reverberate globally. The World Economic Forum projects that the

## *FIGURE 7: POPULATION DISTRIBUTIONS FOR LOW- AND MIDDLE-INCOME COUNTRIES BY REGION*

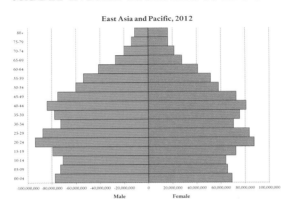

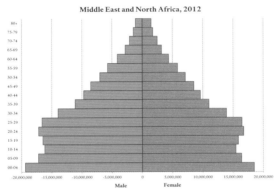

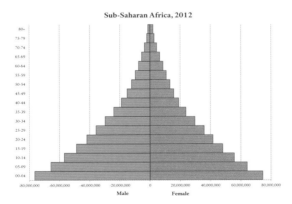

*Data Source:* World Bank, World Development Indicators.

## FIGURE 7: POPULATION DISTRIBUTIONS FOR LOW- AND MIDDLE-INCOME COUNTRIES BY REGION, CONT.

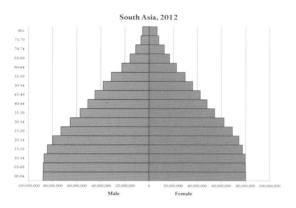

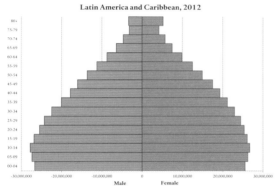

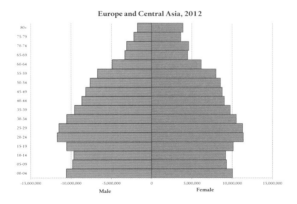

NCD epidemic will inflict $21.3 trillion in economic losses in low- and middle-income countries over the next two decades, which is nearly the same as the total gross domestic product (GDP) of these countries ($24.5 trillion) in 2013.[22]

# The Factors Behind
# the Rising NCD Epidemic

The reasons for the rising NCD epidemic in low- and middle-income countries begin, paradoxically, with increased life expectancy. Better dissemination of breastfeeding and hand-washing information and other low-cost improvements in birth and antenatal care have saved millions of newborn lives. International agencies and donor-funded institutions, such as UNICEF and the Global Alliance for Vaccines and Immunization (GAVI), have extended immunizations for measles, polio, and childhood diseases to the world's poorest. Oral rehydration salts have prevented many of the deaths in children that once occurred in developing countries from cholera and diarrheal disease.[23] Spurred by gains in child health, life expectancies increased, on average, by six months per year in low-income countries between 2000 and 2012.[24] In lower-middle-income countries, the improvement in longevity has been slower, but still impressive: three months annually over the same time.

Longer lives and increased survival beyond adolescence explain why more people in low- and middle-income countries get NCDs. This does not, however, explain why so many people in these countries are developing NCDs so much younger and with such worse outcomes than in wealthier nations.

Part of the answer is that life expectancies have increased in low- and middle-income countries without the improvements in health systems that accompanied the rise in longevity in wealthier countries.[25] The health-care systems in most developing countries are still structured for acute care of infectious diseases and maternal and neonatal mortality, not preventive or chronic care.[26] In many of these countries, medicines are still purchased out of pocket and are often beyond the means of poor households.[27]

Health spending by low- and middle-income country governments has tripled over the past twenty years but remains low relative to

*FIGURE 8: LOW- AND MIDDLE-INCOME COUNTRY GOVERNMENT
HEALTH SPENDING BY REGION*

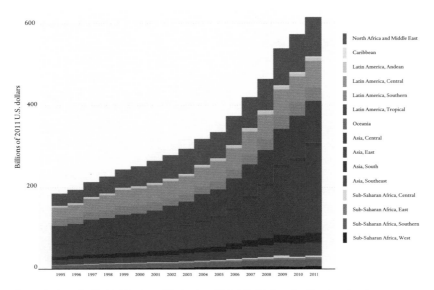

*Source:* Institute for Health Metrics and Evaluation, Global Health Spending Database (2013).

higher-income countries (Figure 8).[28] For instance, all the governments
in sub-Saharan Africa together spend roughly as much on health annually ($33 billion) as the government of Poland ($31 billion).[29] Health
spending by all low- and middle-income country governments, representing 5.7 billion people, is less than is spent by the governments of
Canada, France, Germany, and the United Kingdom, which have a
combined population of 245 million.[30]

The benefits of urbanization, trade, and global integration of
consumer markets to developing countries have been tremendous:
increased food production and distribution, improved hygiene and
sanitation, disseminated medical innovations, lengthened lives, and
millions lifted from abject poverty. Yet these trends have also helped
fuel a rise of NCDs and associated risk factors that is faster than low-
and middle-income countries have been able to establish the health and
regulatory systems necessary to adjust.

Changes in the production, marketing, and distribution of consumer products globally have significantly increased developing countries' exposure to tobacco products, alcohol, and processed food and

beverages. Super- and mega-markets have penetrated every region of the world, even rural areas.[31] Dietary diversity and consumption of fruits and vegetables has declined, especially in East and Southeast Asia and sub-Saharan Africa.[32] Between 1970 and 2000, cigarette consumption tripled in developing countries.[33]

Many developing countries lack the basic consumer protections and public health regulations that have been in place in most high-income countries for decades.[34] The speed and scale of the integration of global consumer markets is overwhelming the little public health infrastructure that does exist in these countries. Developing countries that represent relatively small commercial markets have limited ability to demand labeling and content changes to food, alcohol, and tobacco products produced for global consumption. Multinational corporations may be better resourced than the governments seeking to oversee them.

Tobacco companies, in particular, have used billboards, cartoons, music sponsorships, and other marketing methods long prohibited in developed countries to spur cigarette consumption among women and youths.[35] When countries such as Uruguay, Togo, and Namibia have proposed nondiscriminatory restrictions on cigarette advertising and labeling, multinational tobacco companies have used dispute resolution under trade and investment agreements to block or delay implementation.[36] These tactics have helped raise tobacco sales across Asia, eastern Europe, and Latin America, and many expect them to do so in Africa.

At the same time, low- and middle-income countries are urbanizing at an unprecedented rate. It took fifty years for the world's urban population to increase from 220 million to 732 million in 1950. By 2008, more than half of the global population lived in cities, and the world's urban population is expected to reach almost five billion (60 percent of all people) by 2030.[37] The vast majority of this urbanization is occurring in developing countries and in cities with fewer than one million residents.[38] China and India have the largest urban populations; cities in Africa are growing the fastest.[39]

The urbanization of small- and medium-size cities in developing countries is occurring without the improvements in economic growth or public health infrastructure that accompanied urbanization in wealthier settings.[40] The result has been slums—90 percent of which are in developing countries—that house nearly one billion people.[41] The inhabitants of these densely packed areas, who face pollution outdoors and the burning of fuels indoors, are more susceptible to chronic respiratory diseases. Slum dwellers buy more tobacco products and cheap processed foods and are less likely to have access to adequate nutrition or public-health education.

As a result of these trends, the dominant health risks in low- and middle-income countries have changed (Table 2).[42] Nearly a quarter of the under-age-sixty deaths in developing countries in 2010 are attributed to high blood pressure, smoking, and dietary risks (primarily inadequate intake of fruits, vegetables, and nuts).

TABLE 2: LEADING HEALTH RISKS IN LOW- AND MIDDLE-INCOME COUNTRIES

|    | 1990 | 2010 |
|----|------|------|
| 1. | Childhood underweight | Dietary |
| 2. | Household air pollution | High blood pressure |
| 3. | Suboptimal breast feeding | Smoking |
| 4. | Dietary | Household air pollution |
| 5. | Smoking | Childhood underweight |

Data Source: Institute for Health Metrics and Evaluation, Global Burden of Disease Study 2010.

With little access to preventive care and increased exposure to behavioral risks, working-age people in low- and middle-income countries are more likely to develop an NCD. Without access to chronic care and limited resources, these people are more likely to become disabled and die young as a result of their disease.

In low-income countries, NCDs disproportionately affect the emerging middle class. This population has increased exposure to the health risks associated with NCDs but insufficient resources for the out-of-pocket health services to prevent or treat these diseases. In many lower-middle-income countries, premature NCD death and disability is increasingly associated with poverty, just as it is in high-income countries.[43]

With the trends underlying the emerging NCD crisis in low- and middle-income countries expected to persist or accelerate, the impact of these diseases on working-age populations in these countries will increase. While the share of NCD-related deaths in adults under sixty will continue to fall in higher-income countries, many developing countries are expected to see substantial increases (Figure 9).

FIGURE 9: PREMATURE (UNDER AGE SIXTY) DEATHS FROM NCDS

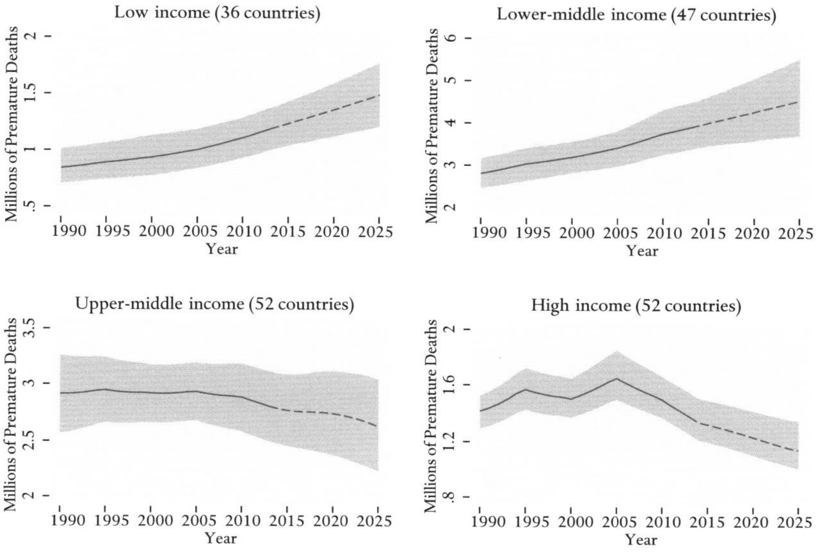

*Underlying Data Source:* Institute for Health Metrics and Evaluation, Global Burden of Disease Study 2013.

The increase will be fastest in sub-Saharan Africa, South Asia, and North Africa and the Middle East, where the rates of working-age NCD-related deaths will grow by 28 percent, 15 percent, and 12 percent by 2025, respectively.[44] Premature death from NCDs such as breast cancer, cardiovascular disease, and lung cancer will increasingly happen in poor countries alone.[45] Overall, under-age-sixty deaths from NCDs in low- and lower- middle-income countries are projected to rise by more than 18 percent, to six million by 2025.[46]

# Current Investments in Addressing NCDs in Developing Countries

The last time that the world confronted a global health challenge that caused such a large number of premature adult deaths and so disproportionately affected low- and middle-income countries was HIV/AIDS. The United States led the global response to that disease, and the world rallied to its side. The U.S. government worked with intergovernmental institutions, donor countries, and philanthropic partners to establish the Global Fund to Fight AIDS, Tuberculosis (TB), and Malaria in 2002 and launched the President's Emergency Plan for AIDS Relief (PEPFAR) in 2003. Together, these programs have delivered life-saving antiretroviral treatments (ARVs) to millions and saved many lives. Competition and voluntary price cuts reduced the per-person cost of these medicines in poor countries from twelve thousand dollars per year in 1999 to two hundred dollars per year in 2003.[47] Funding surged for research and development (R&D) of vaccines, prevention tools, and new and more effective combinations of ARVs.

Since President George W. Bush launched the PEPFAR program in 2003, the United States has committed significant resources to improving health in low- and middle-income countries. Despite the 2008 financial crisis and heated political debates over U.S. government spending, support for global health has remained strong, bipartisan, and one of the hallmarks of U.S. leadership internationally (Figure 10). U.S. engagement in global health has continued to increase under President Barack Obama and with the 2009 launch of the Global Health Initiative (GHI). In 2013, the U.S. Congress reauthorized and appropriated $6.7 billion for PEPFAR and the Global Fund, the highest level of funding in three years.[48]

The U.S. government has invested in nearly eighty countries to provide proven interventions on wide-ranging global health challenges from malaria and tuberculosis to family planning and maternal and child health. Through these programs, the United States has saved

FIGURE 10: U.S. GLOBAL HEALTH PROGRAMS BUDGET,
FY 2001–FY 2014

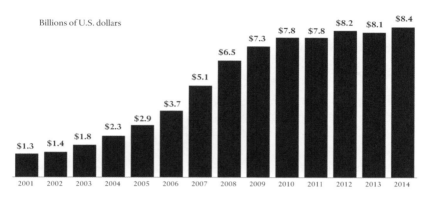

Source: Adapted from Wexler and Kates (March 2014).[49]

millions of lives and inspired the contributions of other governments and philanthropic donors around the world. It is an accomplishment that represents the very best that the United States has to offer and one of which every American may feel deeply proud.

## U.S. RESPONSE TO NCDS

The U.S. response to NCDs, to date, has been modest. It currently has no dedicated programs or budget to address these diseases in low- and middle-income countries.[50] Most U.S. contributions have been spillover benefits of international programs not specifically directed at NCDs, such as investment in primary health care in Haiti, research collaborations and public-private partnerships, and small-scale, ad hoc initiatives to integrate NCD-related objectives into larger existing U.S. global health initiatives.

The following list contains examples of recent and current U.S. interventions on NCDs internationally. This list is meant to be illustrative and may not be exhaustive.

- The U.S. Centers for Disease Control and Prevention (CDC) participates in the Global Tobacco Surveillance System (GTSS) and has advised developing-country governments on cervical cancer

screening, surveillance, and prevention programs.[51] The CDC is col-
laborating with the Pan American Health Organization (PAHO) on
the Global Standardized Hypertension Treatment Project, which aims
to standardize the pharmacological treatment of hypertension in order
to ease its international adoption and improve control rates.[52]

- The U.S. Department of State and the CDC Foundation support the Pink Ribbon Red Ribbon initiative, which leverages the
PEPFAR program to promote breast cancer education and expand
cervical cancer screening and treatment.[53] Private donors and philanthropic entities such as the George W. Bush Institute, Susan G.
Komen Foundation, and the Bill & Melinda Gates Foundation provide most of the programmatic and administrative funding for this
program. PEPFAR also provides support and technical expertise and
helps manage the program.[54]

- The U.S. Department of State, the Environmental Protection Agency,
and ten other U.S. agencies support the Global Alliance for Clean
Cookstoves, a public-private partnership that works to reduce indoor
air pollution.[55] U.S. agencies have provided $67 million in funding to
twenty-five projects, roughly five of which are health related.[56]

- The National Institutes of Health (NIH) funds research on cancer,
diabetes, and NCDs generally. These research programs do not target
these particular needs of developing countries as a general matter,
but may have spillover benefits for global prevention and treatment
of these diseases.

- NIH's National Heart, Lung, and Blood Institute (NHLBI) and Unit-
edHealth Group began the Global Alliance for Chronic Diseases, an
international public-private partnership that facilitates and supports
NCD-related research collaborations via a network of eleven centers
in thirty countries.[57]

- NIH's National Cancer Institute (NCI) has provided trainings on
establishing cancer registries in low- and middle-income countries
and contributed limited support to several sub-Saharan African
countries to do so. NCI promotes U.S. research collaborations with
China and five Latin American countries, participates in the Middle
East Cancer Consortium, provides a four-week training course in
cancer prevention, and offers a small number of grants ($75,000 to
$350,000 each) to South African and Indian researchers working on
low-cost cancer-related technology.[58]

- Between 2002 and 2012, NIH's Fogarty International Center gave $37 million in grants for tobacco control research and capacity building in low- and middle-income countries. In 2012, the Fogarty Center provided $14 million in grants to fifteen international institutions to fund training in NCD-related research.[59] It also supports bilateral scientist exchanges, workshops, and training under the NIH Visiting Program, some of which may be related to developing countries and NCDs.

- The U.S. Agency for International Development (USAID) has provided support for the Global Alliance for Clean Cookstoves, the Uganda Cancer Institute, and a small number of country programs, primarily in eastern Europe and Central Asia, that incorporate NCD-related objectives.[60]

- The Millennium Challenge Corporation has integrated NCD-related goals into at least one of its compact countries.[61]

Assessing the resources dedicated to these NCD-related efforts is difficult because they are generally objectives added to existing U.S. global health programs and not budgeted for separately. The Institute for Health Metrics and Evaluation (IHME) tracks development assistance for global health, and according to its data, the U.S. government dedicated $10.8 million of its more than $8 billion global health aid budget to NCDs in 2010.[62] These aid figures do not include R&D for either communicable or noncommunicable diseases.

## INTERNATIONAL ENGAGEMENT ON NCDS

In the absence of U.S. leadership, the international response to NCDs has struggled. The WHO began issuing reports in the mid-1990s that NCDs would soon dwarf the burden of infectious diseases and maternal, perinatal, and nutritional conditions in developing countries and that the speed and scale of that transition would pose serious challenges to health-care systems and economies.[63] After WHO-issued global strategies and action plans failed to gain traction, a group of concerned low- and middle-income countries and NGOs pressed the United Nations (UN) General Assembly to hold a high-level meeting on NCDs, which occurred in 2011. It is the only health issue other than HIV/AIDS on which the UN General Assembly has held such a meeting.

*FIGURE 11: INTERNATIONAL NCD DEVELOPMENT ASSISTANCE, 2009–2011 PER DALY*

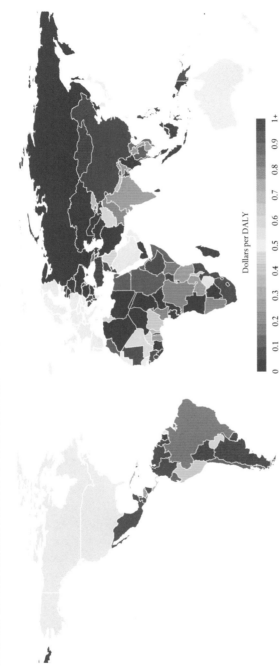

Dollars per DALY

0   0.1   0.2   0.3   0.4   0.5   0.6   0.7   0.8   0.9   1+

*Source:* Institute for Health Metrics and Evaluation, Development Assistance for Health (DAH) database, 2013; Global Burden of Disease Study 2010.[68]

The 2011 UN meeting helped broaden public recognition of the human and economic toll of NCDs and inspired several important country-led initiatives.[64] In May 2012, the WHO set a voluntary global target for reducing premature NCD mortality by 25 percent by 2025, reached agreement with its member states on an international monitoring framework, and released another global action plan on NCDs. More than seventy countries have sought WHO assistance to expand their health-care coverage and cope with the rise of NCDs.[65] To support these efforts, the WHO increased its budget on NCDs by nearly 20 percent, to $318 million.[66] The NCD Alliance, launched in 2009, has helped mobilize more than two thousand organizations to elevate NCDs on the global health agenda. Yet donor aid (Figure 11), in-country resources, and a practical, well-prioritized agenda for collective action on NCDs remain elusive.[67]

# The Case for Increased U.S. Engagement

This Task Force recommends that the U.S. government designate the prevention, diagnosis, and treatment of NCDs in low- and middle-income countries as a priority in its global health and development programs. This is not a recommendation that the Task Force has come to lightly. The resources that the United States has to devote to global health are limited, and its existing commitments are many. The U.S. government is already the largest funder of global health and understandably wary to expand into new areas. With widespread concerns over the U.S. budget and fiscal situation, these are not auspicious times for new initiatives. The Obama administration has indicated an intention to sustain, but not increase, U.S. global health aid.[69]

This recommendation is the unavoidable conclusion of a sober and data-driven assessment of U.S. interests in addressing the rising NCD epidemic in developing countries and the availability of proven, scalable interventions. Through these interventions, the United States may accomplish much while spending relatively little. In this chapter of the report, the Task Force outlines its assessment of U.S. interests in increased engagement on NCDs in low- and middle-income countries and the reasons for doing so now. The following chapter will identify and recommend low-cost strategies for increased U.S. engagement.

## U.S. GLOBAL HEALTH INTERESTS IN NCDS

The United States has two compelling global health interests in increasing its engagement on NCDs. First, NCDs undermine the effectiveness of existing U.S. global health investments. Second, NCDs represent an opportunity for the U.S. government to build on existing U.S. global health platforms to achieve sustainable reductions in premature death and disability that disproportionately affect the poor.

## ENSURING THE EFFECTIVENESS
## OF U.S. GLOBAL HEALTH INVESTMENTS

Surveys have consistently shown that Americans' support for global health depends not on the disease the United States seeks to address, but on the people helped and the effectiveness of aid given.[70] Over the past decade, the U.S. government has invested in addressing HIV/AIDS, TB, and other health challenges facing the poor in dozens of countries and saved millions of lives doing so. Yet the health needs of these countries are changing. The success of U.S. global health efforts cannot continue without changing also.

This Task Force finds that NCDs undermine the effectiveness of U.S. global health investments by causing premature death and disability in the very same populations that the United States is spending substantial resources to save from other diseases. The lion's share of U.S. global health funding is devoted to addressing HIV/AIDS. In 2013, the United States spent $4.7 billion on HIV/AIDS, primarily for treatment and prevention in low- and middle-income countries. A significant portion of the $1.7 billion that the United States contributes to the Global Fund goes to HIV/AIDS and, to a lesser extent, malaria and TB.

Adults between the ages of fifteen and sixty in low- and middle-income countries represent the vast majority of those living with HIV/AIDS and TB and those most likely to contract these diseases in the future. The median ages of death from HIV/AIDS and TB globally are 38.6 and 52.9, respectively.[71] These are the same populations now experiencing worse health and economic effects from the rising NCD epidemic. Recent research indicates that PEPFAR patients in Africa are suffering increasing rates of NCDs such as chronic respiratory illnesses, renal disease, and cervical cancer.[72] It is poor stewardship of scarce U.S. global health resources to spend substantial resources to save an individual from one preventable and treatable disease while that individual succumbs prematurely to another preventable and treatable disease. This is especially true when there are low-cost, proven interventions—such as controlling hypertension or reducing tobacco use—that would make a difference.

The rising epidemic of NCDs undermines U.S. government investments in other areas of global health as well (Figure 12). Smoking increases the risks of TB infection, drug resistance, and poor treatment outcomes.[73] Diabetes triples the likelihood of developing TB.[74] High

*FIGURE 12: U.S. FY13 GLOBAL HEALTH FUNDING*

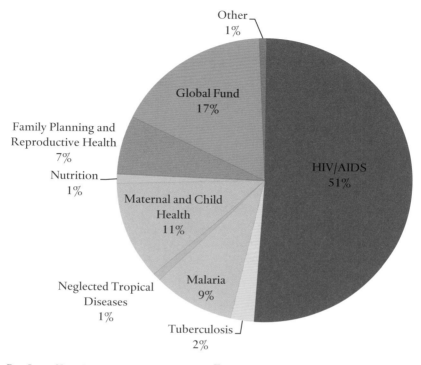

*Data Source:* Henry J. Kaiser Family Foundation, 2014.[77]

blood pressure and gestational diabetes increase adverse pregnancy and maternal health outcomes.[75] People infected with the hepatitis C virus, which causes liver cancer and cirrhosis, are also more likely to develop schistosomiasis than those who are not.[76] More broadly, failure to address the rising epidemic of NCDs undermines the U.S. objective of building sustainable health systems in low- and middle-income countries and their ability to assume ownership of U.S. programs on communicable disease and maternal health.

To assess the potential threat of NCDs to the progress achieved thus far by U.S. global health investments, the Task Force undertook a detailed analysis of the low- and middle-income countries where the U.S. government currently has significant health investments. The analysis assessed the leading health risk factors and the premature (under age sixty) burden of NCDs relative to HIV/AIDS, TB, malaria, and maternal, newborn, and child health (MNCH). The countries assessed include twenty-nine designated as priorities under the GHI[78] as well as twenty other countries that received more than $5 million in U.S. health aid in 2013.[79] The annex to this report includes case studies on each of these forty-nine countries (hereafter "U.S. priority countries").[80]

NCDs are rising in young, working-age populations in these U.S. priority countries and resulting in poor health outcomes. NCDs accounted for 28 percent of the premature deaths and a third of the DALYs in the priority countries in 2010 (Figure 13). These rates are 3.5 times greater than premature deaths and 5.5 times greater than disability attributed to HIV/AIDS in these countries. In the same year, NCDs were responsible for 1.6 times as many premature deaths as malaria, TB, and HIV combined in these priority countries. Four of the five leading health risks in these countries are behavioral and clinical risks for NCDs—diet, indoor air pollution, tobacco smoking, and high blood pressure.

The health outcomes for those who develop NCDs in these forty-nine U.S. priority countries are poor (Figure 14). In recent years, women and

*FIGURE 13: CAUSE OF HEALTH BURDEN IN U.S. PRIORITY COUNTRIES*

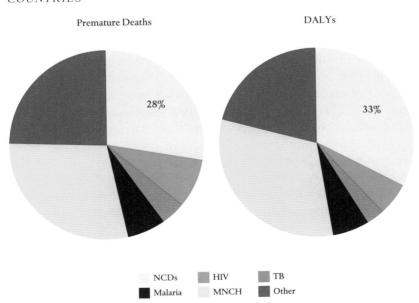

Premature Deaths

DALYs

28%

33%

NCDs    HIV    TB
Malaria    MNCH    Other

*Data Source:* Institute for Health Metrics and Evaluation, Global Burden of Disease Study 2010.

*FIGURE 14: AGE-ADJUSTED NCD RATES FOR U.S. PRIORITY COUNTRIES*

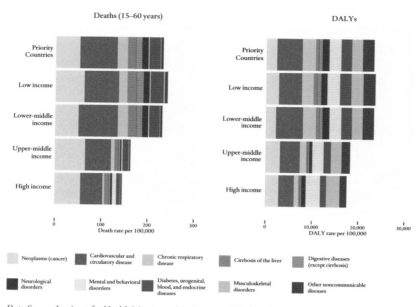

*Data Source:* Institute for Health Metrics and Evaluation, Global Burden of Disease Study 2010.

children have been a particular focus of these U.S. global health investments. The health outcomes are particularly bad for women and girls who have one or more NCD in these priority countries; in 2010, they had an 83 percent higher age-standard death rate than in high-income countries.[81] These outcomes reflect the disproportionate challenge that NCDs represent to women and children in developing countries. Women in these settings often lack control over household resources and hence have less access to diagnosis, prevention, and care for NCDs for themselves and their children. Ninety-two percent of the cases of hyperglycemia (high blood glucose) in pregnancy occur in developing countries, mostly to women unaware of their condition or its elevated risks for obstructed labor and preeclampsia.[82] Acute rheumatic fever is a leading cause of cardiovascular disease in sub-Saharan Africa, mostly affects youth, and is generally caused by delayed or inadequate treatment of strep infections in children.[83]

On a national level, NCDs will deplete scarce health-care resources in these priority countries, making it harder for those governments struggling to address still-high rates of childhood malnutrition and infectious diseases such as TB and HIV/AIDS. In doing so, preventable and premature deaths and disability from NCDs diminish the value of the U.S. investments in building sustainable health systems in poor countries.

### LEVERAGING EXISTING U.S. GLOBAL HEALTH INVESTMENTS TO REDUCE THE BURDEN OF PREVENTABLE AND PREMATURE DEATHS DUE TO NCDS

NCDs are similar to many existing U.S. global health priorities. As with prenatal and maternal care, family planning, nutrition, and reproductive health care, the health of U.S. citizens does not directly depend on reducing NCDs abroad. And as with HIV/AIDS, which is transmitted primarily through unprotected sex and intravenous drug use, most of the risk factors for NCDs are behavioral, such as tobacco use and indoor pollution. Roughly half of the countries that received $5 million or more in U.S. health assistance in 2013 were lower-middle- or middle-income countries, and it is in these same countries that the burden of NCDs is the greatest.[84] But the most important way in which NCDs are similar to other U.S. global health priorities is that these diseases cause significant amounts of preventable and premature death and disability among the poor that U.S. leadership could help sustainably reduce.

U.S. leadership in global health is a rare area of political consensus in increasingly partisan times. The durability of that leadership in global health reflects American values—compassion, charity, and a willingness to share U.S. technological advances in disease prevention, diagnosis, and treatment with the poor who need them.[85] By doing so, the United States affords millions of underserved and vulnerable people the opportunity to lead healthy and productive lives. In deciding to approve the proposal for the PEPFAR program, President George W. Bush reportedly asked how the United States would be judged if it did not act to address a preventable and treatable epidemic of such magnitude.[86]

The analysis of the forty-nine U.S. priority countries where the United States has significant global health investments demonstrates that NCDs are the dominant, fast-emerging challenge facing the poor, underserved, and vulnerable in these settings. Established U.S. programs in these countries to address HIV/AIDS, TB, and maternal and child health offer an existing platform for NCD prevention, screening, and treatment. Relatively inexpensive opportunities abound.

A decade into PEPFAR, the U.S. government has developed extensive experience supporting quality care for chronic conditions in resource-poor settings. PEPFAR is the largest chronic-care program in many low- and middle-income countries. NCD prevention and treatment strategies incorporate similar elements of management of HIV/AIDS: promotion of healthy behaviors, long-term adherence to prescribed treatment, consistent monitoring of treatment outcomes, and patient engagement in care and treatment decisions.[87] The same approaches that the U.S. government uses to ensure safe, reliable supplies of AIDS and malaria treatment, childhood vaccines, and contraceptives could be leveraged to improve access to the essential and generally off-patent medicines needed to address NCDs in developing countries. U.S. nutrition programs targeting the first one thousand days of life can simultaneously help address NCDs. Increasing evidence shows low-birth-weight babies who gain weight rapidly in childhood suffer greater risks of hypertension and diabetes later in life.[88]

There are existing examples of successful NCD programs that leverage HIV/AIDS program platforms. Integration of HIV/AIDS, diabetes, and hypertension management in Cambodia has demonstrated high acceptance and good outcomes.[89] A successful low-technology screen-and-treat program for cervical cancer in women with HIV was piloted through PEPFAR in Zambia.[90] A clinic in Uganda uses the same staff and systems to offer services for HIV on some days and for diabetes and heart disease during the remainder of the week.[91] PEPFAR has integrated other global health objectives such as family and reproductive care, maternal health, and nutrition into its programs and platforms.[92] More research is needed to ensure integration of NCD objectives is cost-effective, does not diminish the effectiveness of HIV-related programming, and reaches the target patient population—men—as well as women and children.

## U.S. ECONOMIC AND STRATEGIC INTERESTS IN ADDRESSING NCDS

Speaking before the United Nations, President Obama cited global health as not only a moral objective but also a U.S. strategic and economic imperative.[93] The 2000 U.S. National Intelligence Estimate, titled *The Global Infectious Disease Threat and Its Implications for the United States*, likewise recognized the importance of global health to the achievement of these foreign policy and trade objectives.[94] These conclusions have been reaffirmed and reinforced in the 2010 U.S. National Security Strategy, the U.S. State Department's 2012 Quadrennial Diplomacy and Development Review, and National Intelligence Council reports.[95]

The Task Force finds that the United States has two compelling strategic interests in increasing its engagement on NCDs. First, the United States has an important interest in fostering the long-term capacity of low- and middle-income countries to prevent and reduce premature NCD-related death and disability as a means of supporting economic development and promoting U.S. exports. Second, the United States has interests in enhancing the credibility of U.S. global health programs and building fruitful partnerships with capable allies and rising powers.

## U.S. ECONOMIC INTERESTS IN ADDRESSING NCDS

U.S. global health investments help expand the ranks of prosperous and capable states, particularly in Africa; build a more stable, inclusive global economy; and unleash the potential of previously impoverished and vulnerable populations. In doing so, the United States advances its own interests in international trade, U.S. exports, and American jobs.

Ninety-five percent of the world's customers and 75 percent of global purchasing power now reside beyond U.S. borders. Developing countries have represented roughly half of global growth since the 2008 financial crisis.[96] U.S. private-sector investments in sub-Saharan Africa over the past decade have yielded among the highest rates of return of any region in the world.[97] In 2013, the United States exported $706 billion in goods and services to low- and middle-income countries.[98] As developing countries become wealthier, their demand for exports is expected to grow and shift to the categories in which the United States leads the world: civilian aircraft, pharmaceuticals, machinery and equipment, high-value foods, and entertainment.[99]

NCDs undermine the continued prosperity of low- and middle-income countries. Few other threats can compare with the human and economic toll that NCDs are projected to exact in these countries. The frequent onset of NCDs among young people and the bad health outcomes that result have devastating economic and social consequences (Figure 15). The chronic nature of most of these diseases means patients are sick and suffer longer and they seek and require more medical care and hospitalization.

*FIGURE 15: PROPORTION OF NCD DALYS AMONG ALL DALYS
BY AGE*

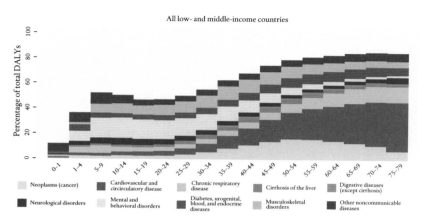

*Data Source:* Institute for Health Metrics and Evaluation, Global Burden of Disease Study 2010.

In low-income countries, the risk of premature NCD death and disability is highest among the emerging middle class. Low-income countries cannot sustain economic growth unless their middle-class and working-age people survive. In many lower- and middle-income countries, premature NCD death and disability is increasingly associated with poverty, just as it is in high-income countries.[100] The World Economic Forum has ranked NCDs as a greater threat to global economic development than fiscal crises, natural disasters, and transnational crime and corruption.[101]

## U.S. STRATEGIC INTERESTS IN ADDRESSING NCDS

U.S. investments in global health are visible, concrete, and highly valued; they save lives and have enhanced U.S. credibility around the world.[102] Although U.S. generosity on HIV/AIDS, maternal and child health, and other global health challenges will always be valued, it will be increasingly difficult to justify—to both U.S. taxpayers and aid recipients—such a disproportionately small share going to the diseases and risk factors that cause the majority of preventable death and suffering in the working-age poor in the countries where U.S. investments occur.

In the forty-nine U.S. priority countries, IHME data indicates that the U.S. government spent in 2010 $44.17 in aid per each DALY lost to

HIV/AIDS, $4.21 for each DALY lost to malaria, and $1.41 per maternal, child, and nutritional health DALY, but $0.02 for each DALY lost to
NCDs.[103] The discrepancies in U.S. global health spending will grow in
the coming years as the NCD crisis expands in low- and middle-income
countries—particularly in South Asia and sub-Saharan Africa—and
continues to afflict young people disproportionately.

Global health has also long been and remains one of the important
ways in which the United States advances its foreign policy interests in a
just and sustainable international order that fosters peace, stability, and
cooperation on meeting global challenges.[104] The U.S. National Intelligence Estimate in 2000 was the first to consider these strategic interests
in the context of nontraditional health threats:

> Chronic, noncommunicable diseases; neglected tropical diseases;
> maternal and child mortality; malnutrition; sanitation and access
> to clean water; and availability of basic health care also affect the
> U.S. national interest through their effects on the economies, gov-
> ernments, and militaries of key countries and regions.[105]

The FY 2013 distribution of development assistance reflects U.S. strategic interests in countries, but not yet in the NCDs or other nontraditional health threats that these countries face. Substantial U.S. aid went
to address health challenges in strategically important countries such as
Afghanistan, Jordan, Lebanon, India, Pakistan, Ukraine, Indonesia, and
Vietnam.[106] Smaller amounts of U.S. health assistance, between $1 mil-
lion and $4 million, supported health programs in Brazil, China, Egypt,
Georgia, and Thailand in FY 2013.[107]

The premature burden of NCDs in all these countries dwarfs the
rates of HIV/AIDS, malaria, TB, and the other current targets of U.S.
health programs. The World Bank, for example, estimates that one-
third of people in Ukraine die before the age of sixty-five, overwhelm-
ingly from NCDs.[108] Another World Bank study concluded that NCDs
reduce the labor supply in Egypt by approximately 19 percent, at a loss
of roughly 12 percent of GDP.[109] The prevalence of NCDs is staggering
in India and China and growing rapidly in Brazil, Indonesia, and Pakistan (Table 3).

NCDs and their associated health-care costs are a pressing concern
for the economies and governments of countries of U.S. strategic interest and an important, untapped opportunity for collaboration. This is

particularly true in the emerging nations where NCDs are starting to
strain institutional capacity and spur political instability. Concerns over
the health effects of environmental pollution and inadequate health-
care systems have already led to mass protests in China and Brazil.[110]
As the NCD epidemic expands, the economic costs of these diseases
on working-age people and households could escalate into popular dissatisfaction with the governments in other countries and regions where
U.S. interests lie.

TABLE 3: COUNTRIES WITH THE LARGEST NCD BURDEN

|  | Premature NCD deaths | NCD DALYs |
|---|---|---|
| 1. | India (1.7 million) | China (244 million) |
| 2. | China (1.6 million) | India (236 million) |
| 3. | Russia (0.4 million) | Russia (48 million) |
| 4. | Indonesia (0.3 million) | Indonesia (45 million) |
| 5. | Pakistan (0.2 million) | Brazil (38 million) |

Data Source: Institute for Health Metrics and Evaluation, Global Burden of Disease Study 2010.

### U.S. INTERESTS IN ADDRESSING NCDS NOW

The Task Force finds that the United States has strong interests in not
only increasing its engagement on the rising NCD epidemic in developing countries, but in doing so now. The costs of child and adult health
are diverging in low- and lower-middle-income countries (Figure 16).[111]
Even poor countries are achieving the low child mortality rates that
were once only possible in wealthy countries. The opposite is true for
adults; the economic growth that developing countries must sustain just
to achieve the health performance that existed in developed countries
more than sixty years ago has risen sharply since the mid-1990s. Those
trends are independent of HIV/AIDS—a variable for which Figure 16
controls—and occur despite dramatic declines in communicable diseases over the same time period. NCDs are the reason.

Three conclusions emerge from this analysis. First, effectively
addressing NCDs in low- and lower-middle-income countries is likely
to become more difficult with each passing year of inaction. Second,

FIGURE 16: GDP PER CAPITA ASSOCIATED WITH LOW- AND
LOWER-MIDDLE-INCOME COUNTRIES ACHIEVING THE MEDIAN
MORTALITY RATES THAT EXISTED IN HIGH-INCOME COUNTRIES
IN 1950

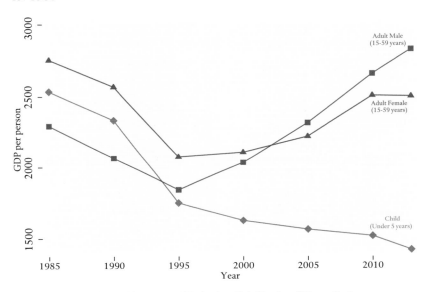

*Data Source:* Institute for Health Metrics and Evaluation, Global Burden of Disease Study 2013.

economic growth alone is unlikely to solve the NCD crisis in most of
these countries. Fewer developing countries will be able to keep pace
with the fast-growing costs of the NCD epidemic, particularly as working-age adults (ages fifteen to fifty-nine) begin to represent the majority
of their populations. Third, effective, relatively low-cost international
initiatives can make a difference, as they have with child health. U.S.
programs on immunization, oral rehydration, and birth and antenatal
care have contributed to the dramatic improvement in child and infant
health in poor countries over the past twenty years.

   There are time-limited opportunities for the United States to work
with partner countries and donors to help prevent critical expansions in
the NCD epidemic. For example, tobacco-use rates in Africa are relatively low but projected to increase.[112] Personal income and consumer
spending are rising, and the populations in the region are young.[113]
Youths in many of these countries are beginning to smoke earlier than
in past generations, sometimes at age eight or nine.[114] Many African

governments have not yet implemented effective tobacco control programs. The American Cancer Society projects that, unless urgent action
is taken, Africa will have the second-most smokers of any region by
2060.[115] Many African governments lack the health-care resources and
infrastructure to cope with the epidemic of tobacco-related diseases
that would result.[116] Timely U.S. leadership can help countries avoid
that outcome.

The United States also has an opportunity to leverage the September 2015 announcement of the UN Sustainable Development Goals
(SDGs), which will succeed the Millennium Development Goals
(MDGs) when they expire in 2015. The SDGs are expected to include
objectives on reducing premature NCD-related deaths by one-third
by 2030 and strengthening implementation of the WHO Framework
Convention on Tobacco Control.[117] With U.S. leadership and support, these objectives could play a similar catalytic role as the MDGs,
which many credit with helping inspire the rapid increase in international aid to address HIV/AIDS, malaria, and maternal and child
health.[118] The SDGs also correspond well to the strategy and recommendations for U.S. engagement on NCDs that are outlined in the
next section of this report.

# How the United States Can Make a Difference

Even when limited to the four diseases causing the majority of the NCD burden in low- and middle-income countries, cancers, cardiovascular diseases, chronic respiratory illnesses, and diabetes involve a wide range of risk factors and potential prevention and treatment strategies. Stemming the rise of these diseases will require developing countries to retool their health-care systems to provide preventive and chronic care, improve urban design, and maintain effective regulatory, agricultural, and public health systems. These are challenges that high-income countries share, including the United States. The difference is that demographic and economic changes are forcing developing countries to confront those challenges faster and with fewer resources.

Determining health priorities and allocating resources in the face of the emerging NCD epidemic are decisions for national governments. Yet the direction of those decisions is deeply influenced by the priorities of the United States, as are the priorities of the other donor governments, nongovernmental organizations, and philanthropic institutions that compose the global health community. U.S. support for cost-effective NCD programs would reduce preventable death and disability, demonstrate the feasibility of doing so, and raise expectations and accountability for local governments and other global health actors.

The Task Force finds that increased engagement on the rising epidemic of NCDs is vital to U.S. interests—in improved global health, increased international trade and development, and U.S. standing and strategic objectives around the world. The Task Force also finds that, conversely, U.S. leadership can make an enormous difference in helping developing countries meet the NCD challenge, but the role for U.S. intervention is necessarily limited to the areas and activities in which it may be effective.

## A STRATEGY FOR U.S. ENGAGEMENT

This Task Force has been asked to recommend practical, scalable ways that the U.S. government can work with like-minded partners to help address the rising NCD epidemic in low- and middle-income countries, even in these austere times. We have come together on a strategy and a set of concrete recommendations that we believe offers the broad outline of a workable way forward.

The Task Force recommends that U.S. investments in NCDs should focus initially on the specific NCDs and risk factors that are (a) especially prevalent among working-age populations of the developing-country poor and for which (b) effective and low-cost interventions exist that are (c) amenable to collective action and (d) can leverage existing U.S. programs and platforms. These efforts should be country-specific and designed in cooperation with the local government to be responsive to its needs, interests, and capacities. U.S. interventions should be rigorously and transparently monitored to maintain congressional and public support and, if proven cost-effective, to promote their broader adoption by low- and middle-income countries. Where possible, U.S. efforts should leverage regional platforms, which would promote knowledge sharing and technical capacity of other countries not directly targeted by U.S. NCD investments.

We have applied these criteria to the specific diseases and health risks that are causing large numbers of premature deaths in low- and middle-income countries but far fewer in high-income countries due to the widespread availability of effective prevention and treatment measures. In large part, it is these diseases and risks that are responsible for the divergence in the NCD epidemics in developed and developing countries. Assessment of these diseases and risk factors provides the basis for this Task Force's recommendations in three categories: challenges on which U.S. leadership could make a tremendous difference on NCDs now; challenges on which U.S. leadership could make a tremendous difference in the near term; and shared challenges on which increased U.S. collaboration with developing-country governments and the private sector may yield cost-effective ideas of mutual benefit.

# NCD Challenges on Which U.S. Leadership Would Make a Difference Now

The Task Force recommends actions to address four challenges on which U.S. engagement would make a difference now and meet the selection criteria outlined earlier. Each challenge is especially prevalent among working-age populations in the low- and middle-income countries where the United States has existing platforms for action. Low-cost, prevention-based solutions exist for each challenge, and the United States is in the position to help local governments implement them. Each challenge is one on which U.S. leadership would reduce the burden that the rising epidemic of NCDs is posing to governments, economies, and, most important, people in low- and middle-income countries. A brief investment case is provided for each challenge.

## CARDIOVASCULAR DISEASE

Cardiovascular diseases in low- and middle-income countries cause thirteen million deaths each year, more than a quarter of all deaths in these countries. Most of these cardiovascular deaths result from ischemic heart disease, also known as coronary heart disease, and cerebrovascular disease, which produces strokes.[119] These diseases present a substantial and rising threat in the same forty-nine countries where the United States has substantial annual health investments (Figure 17).

### AVAILABILITY OF PROVEN INTERVENTIONS

Given that cardiovascular diseases produce so many NCD-related deaths in developing countries, effective prevention and treatment strategies could save a large number of lives. Fortunately, these strategies exist and are in widespread use in high-income countries. Despite

*FIGURE 17: CHANGE IN PREMATURE CARDIOVASCULAR DEATHS IN U.S. PRIORITY COUNTRIES, 1990–2013*

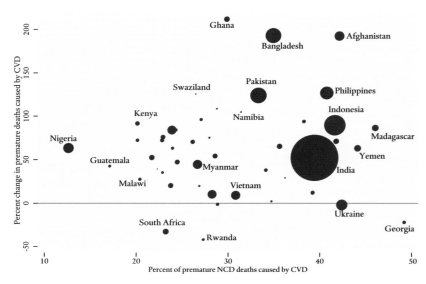

*Data Source:* Institute for Health Metrics and Evaluation, Global Burden of Disease Study 2013.

increasing rates of obesity, the United States cut mortality rates from these diseases by more than 40 percent between 1980 and 2000.[120] Mortality from stroke and coronary heart disease has declined by as much as two-thirds in some high-income countries.[121]

Two factors contributed to this improvement. First, there were substantial declines in smoking, hypertension, and other risk factors in high-income countries. Second, there has been a revolution in the effectiveness of treatments.

Hypertension, also known as high blood pressure, is responsible for an estimated one-half of the global deaths and disability from coronary heart disease and nearly two-thirds of the deaths and disability from stroke worldwide.[122] In parts of Africa, Asia, and eastern Europe, prevalence of high blood pressure exceeds 45 percent.[123] Hypertension control can be achieved using existing and off-patent medications such as diuretics, calcium channel blockers, ACE inhibitors, and beta-blockers. The Institute of Medicine recommends hypertension control programs as an ideal first step for cardiovascular disease prevention and control because the health benefits accrue in a relatively short time. Hypertension management is also a good platform for adding other future prevention objectives on tobacco use and high blood-lipid levels, a risk factor for diabetes.[124]

In adults who have had a previous stroke or heart attack, use of aspirin, beta-blockers, and ACE inhibitors is especially effective. Taken independently, these drugs reduce the risk of reoccurrence of cardiovascular events by about one-quarter; taken in combination, these drugs reduce reoccurrence by two-thirds to three-quarters.[125] Implementing secondary prevention of cardiovascular disease requires a commitment to community surveillance programs and the collection of mortality and morbidity data to identify high-risk individuals.[126] Advanced profiling has been used in the treatment of hypertension in South Africa and found to be a cost-effective means of targeting those at higher risk in resource-poor environments.[127]

### WHAT THE UNITED STATES HAS TO OFFER

The same strategies that U.S. officials employed toward tuberculosis control in New York City and have supported internationally would make a significant contribution to reducing the large premature burden of cardiovascular disease in low- and middle-income countries. These strategies include standardizing and simplifying diagnostic and treatment protocols; ensuring a consistent supply of essential quality-assured medicines; identifying at-risk individuals participating in other health-care services; and systematic monitoring and evaluation of outcomes and patients. This approach has been successfully piloted for hypertension at an HIV clinic in Malawi that treats fifty thousand patients and relies on nurses to provide most of the associated health services.[128]

To make this strategy work on a broader scale, more support should be devoted to scaling CDC collaboration with PAHO on the Global Standardized Hypertension Treatment Project. This program could make a critical contribution to standardizing cost-effective pharmacologic treatment of hypertension, easing its international adoption, and improving high-blood-pressure control rates globally.[129] More resources would allow that process to occur much faster and be implemented in other regions.

ACE inhibitors, beta-blockers, and many statins are off-patent but still unavailable in many developing countries. The recent Prospective Urban Rural Epidemiology (PURE) study found that 69 percent of patients in lower-middle-income countries and 80 percent in low-income countries did not receive these medications at all, compared to only 11 percent of high-income-country patients. Many of these products lack international suppliers or are difficult for still-nascent developing-country regulatory authorities to oversee.[130]

The United States should seek to expand existing procurement and treatment platforms, such as PEPFAR, to include hypertension medicines and help ensure the quality, safety, and consistent supply of these cardiovascular medicines. Assisting the WHO in expanding its prequalification program to NCD medicines would compensate for developing-country regulators who are still unable to register and oversee these products. Development of these procurement and regulatory pathways should engage multilateral and bilateral development agencies, medical societies, public and private payers, pharmaceutical and medical-device companies, and health technology assessment experts to ensure rational use of these technologies.

Another way to address drug availability and affordability is through a combination of generic cardiovascular disease medications known as the polypill. This single intervention would improve patient adherence to treatment regimes, but it requires more clinical research in low-resource settings before it may be used in at-risk populations that have not yet experienced a cardiovascular attack. The United States should support this research and, if it proves successful, promote the rollout of the polypill through global health product procurement platforms.

Finally, the United States should leverage its global health programs to identify patients with a history of heart disease or risk of developing one. Once the most relevant settings are identified, the United States should pilot cost-effective, low-resource hypertension monitoring and treatment programs and build registries. Hypertension registries collect and store clinical information on patients who have the condition and create the evidence base for evaluating the effectiveness of interventions and changes in population needs. Once established for hypertension, these registries may later be expanded to monitor other health risks such as tobacco use and glycemic control.

## COST-EFFECTIVENESS

High blood pressure is a major contributor to both coronary heart disease and stroke. Even small decreases in the incidence of high blood pressure could have a profound effect on lowering cardiovascular disease rates. Aspirin and beta-blocker usage studies have shown them to be highly cost-effective.[131] The Disease Control Priority Network, a collaboration between the World Bank, the Bill & Melinda Gates Foundation, the University of Washington, and other leading health organizations, has determined acute management of heart attacks with low-cost drugs is highly cost-effective, generating twenty-five dollars in health and economic savings for every dollar of investment.

## POTENTIAL IMPACT

The benefits of reducing cardiovascular disease risks are not only large but can be realized within five years. The full benefits of most other NCD interventions, such as smoking cessation, take longer to manifest.[132]

As a rough indication of what is possible with U.S. leadership, the Task Force estimated the expected increase in cardiovascular deaths in the forty-nine U.S. priority countries and the increase that would exist if those countries made improvements at the same rate that the average high-income country did between 2000 and 2013 (Figure 18). The difference between those projections is 3.5 million premature deaths and 14.2 million deaths overall in eleven years in just those priority countries. The projection accounts for the expected demographic changes in each country, such as population growth and aging.

*FIGURE 18: PROJECTED PREMATURE CARDIOVASCULAR DEATHS IN U.S. PRIORITY COUNTRIES, 2014–2025*

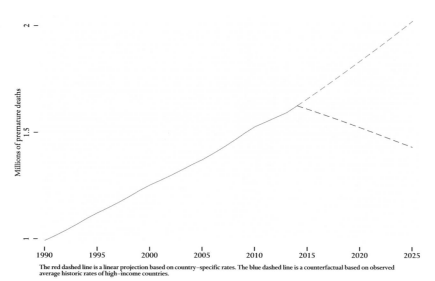

The red dashed line is a linear projection based on country–specific rates. The blue dashed line is a counterfactual based on observed average historic rates of high–income countries.

*Underlying Data Source:* Institute for Health Metrics and Evaluation, Global Burden of Disease Study 2013.

## TOBACCO

Tobacco use is the second leading cause of disease and premature death worldwide, behind hypertension. In response to stagnating sales in high-income nations, multinational companies have targeted low- and middle-income countries with still-limited tobacco tax and regulatory systems.[133] Unless international tobacco control efforts improve, and soon, the WHO projects tobacco-related illnesses will kill eight million people annually by 2030 and one billion by the end of this century, mostly in developing countries.[134]

Figure 19 is a partial indication of the increasing threat that tobacco represents to the same countries wherein the United States has substantial annual health investments. Seventy percent of lung cancer deaths worldwide are due to tobacco use; smokers are twenty times more likely to perish from that disease than nonsmokers.[135] The rise in cigarette smoking has already made lung cancer the most common cancer and cause of death from cancer in low- and middle-income countries.[136]

FIGURE 19: CHANGE IN PREMATURE LUNG CANCER DEATHS IN
U.S. PRIORITY COUNTRIES, 1990–2013

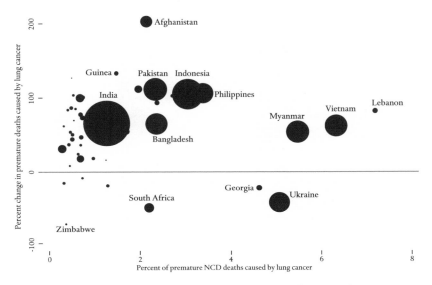

Data Source: Institute for Health Metrics and Evaluation, Global Burden of Disease Study 2013.

Lung cancer is an incomplete measure of the consequences of
tobacco use and secondhand smoke because they are also the leading
risk factors for other cancers and all the major NCDs—diabetes, cardiovascular disease, and respiratory disease.[137] Tobacco use increases
health risks at every stage of life: pregnancy complications, congenital
abnormalities, childhood illnesses, TB infection, drug resistance, poor
treatment outcomes, and increased mortality.[138] Forty percent of the
world's children—700 million—breathe secondhand tobacco smoke at
home and suffer increased rates of asthma and lower-respiratory infections as a result.[139] Stopping smoking can lead to a gain of about ten
years in life expectancy.

### AVAILABILITY OF PROVEN INTERVENTIONS

Tobacco control works. Comprehensive tobacco control programs are
cost-effective and evidence based.[140] A recent review of more than one
hundred econometric studies concluded that tobacco taxes and consumption are strongly inversely correlated, particularly in low- and

middle-income countries.[141] According to the World Bank, each 10 percent increase in the retail price of tobacco products in developing countries reduces tobacco consumption by roughly 8 percent and tobacco use prevalence by about 4 percent.[142] Youths and low-income smokers are more likely to quit in response to price increases.[143] Bans on direct and indirect advertising or promotion of tobacco products, particularly when comprehensive, have likewise been shown to reduce consumption.[144] Strong evidence also exists that bans on smoking in public places reduce exposure to secondhand tobacco smoke and can help decrease overall cigarette consumption.[145]

These strategies have worked in developing and developed countries alike. Higher excise taxes, bans on smoking in public settings, and marketing restrictions combined with the increased stigmatization of tobacco use through public health campaigns and civil suits have more than halved adult smoking rates from 42 percent to 19 percent in the United States since 1965.[146] Mexico, which has long had high cigarette taxes, is one of only four countries worldwide to reduce smoking by more than 50 percent in both men and women since 1980. In 2008, Turkey raised cigarette taxes to 81 percent and banned tobacco advertising and smoking in public places. The following year, hospital emergency room admissions in Turkey for smoking-related disease declined by nearly a quarter and smoking rates dropped 16 percent over three years.[147]

Platforms already exist for establishing and expanding effective tobacco control programs in low- and middle-income countries. The WHO Framework Convention on Tobacco Control (FCTC) provides a blueprint for comprehensive tobacco control by prescribing specific domestic tobacco control strategies to reduce the supply and demand for tobacco products. The FCTC is binding and one of the world's most widely subscribed treaties, with 176 member countries representing more than 90 percent of the world's population.[148] The FCTC entered into force in 2005 and, like nearly all treaties concluded since that time, the U.S. Senate has yet to approve it. The United States has signed the FCTC, however, and is fully compliant with its terms.

In 2008, the WHO, with support from Bloomberg Philanthropies, developed MPOWER, a package of evidence-based and measurable strategies to support FCTC implementation at the country level.[149] In subsequent years, adoption of MPOWER measures on tobacco advertising and health warning labels has improved in low- and middle-income countries, including in the forty-nine U.S. priority countries, but continues to lag in other areas and especially on tobacco taxes.[150]

## WHAT THE UNITED STATES HAS TO OFFER

Tobacco control requires a mix of expertise and inputs—taxation, product regulation, surveillance, and program monitoring and evaluation—that have not historically resided at the WHO or national health ministries. U.S. agencies have that expertise and should work with international partners to provide the technical assistance that low- and middle-income country governments need.

CDC support for international tobacco control surveillance is invaluable and cheap, performed on a budget of $3 million in 2009.[151] This Task Force recommends that the CDC should be appropriated the resources to increase that budget and expand its international tobacco programs to the lowest-income countries, where tobacco use is rising fastest and surveillance data is least reliable.

Implementing effective tobacco taxation is complicated by factors that vary between countries and cultures. These factors include tobacco use prevalence, price elasticity, the availability of counterfeit tobacco products, and earmarking to maintain sustainability of taxation schemes.[152] Some low-income countries lack the capacity and expertise to administer and collect excise taxes. The Task Force recommends that U.S. agencies with the necessary expertise partner with the World Bank and the International Monetary Fund (IMF) to provide technical assistance to interested developing countries on tobacco taxation and suppression of the illicit cigarette trade. This recommendation would build on a successful pilot that Bloomberg Philanthropies and the Bill & Melinda Gates Foundation funded that temporarily placed two CDC tax specialists at the World Bank to help the Philippines, Russia, and other countries implement or increase tobacco taxes.[153]

Product labeling and the regulation of nicotine, tar, and tobacco additives are important components of limiting the public health impact of cigarettes. Most developing countries do not have the regulatory acumen to implement these programs. In 2009, Congress granted the U.S. Food and Drug Administration (FDA) the mandate for tobacco product regulation. It is now one of only a handful of national regulatory agencies with expertise in this area. Congress should expand the resources of the FDA to work with interested developing countries to implement tobacco product regulations pursuant to the FCTC.

The opportunities to leverage U.S. global health platforms exist. The Task Force supports the integration of tobacco education and cessation into U.S. maternal and child health and TB initiatives. These programs engage populations at risk for tobacco use, particularly girls in developing countries.

Finally, the Obama administration has announced its intention to safeguard tobacco control laws and regulations from unnecessary trade and investment challenges under the Trans-Pacific Partnership, a pending trade deal between the United States and eleven other countries. The Task Force believes that this announcement provides an important opportunity to forge an appropriate balance of U.S. trade and global health priorities. The Task Force urges the Obama administration to negotiate an exception that encompasses the full range of nondiscriminatory tobacco control measures addressed under the FCTC and permitted under U.S. law.[154]

### AVAILABLE COST ESTIMATES

Improved tobacco control is first among WHO "best buy" strategies for addressing NCDs. It is cost-effective and, due to its emphasis on taxation, revenue generating. The Disease Control Priority Network estimates comprehensive tobacco control programs in developing countries also generate a return of forty-to-one in health-care costs saved.

Yet tobacco control programs do require resources to establish. This Task Force recommends that the United States work with other donors to create a multi-donor trust fund at the World Bank, which would provide seed funding to interested low-income countries to institute and enforce tobacco tax legislation until it becomes self-sustaining. The Bill & Melinda Gates Foundation established a similar World Bank trust fund to support global medicines' regulatory harmonization with $12.5 million over five years, which has been successful and subsequently supported by the United Kingdom and PEPFAR.[155]

Doubling the current $3 million CDC budget for international tobacco control surveillance would be low cost but would help generate the timely, accurate data that governments and donors need to address increased tobacco use in low-income countries. The other recommendations of this Task Force on tobacco would likewise be relatively cheap—mostly staffing, travel, and funding for pilot projects to integrate tobacco control into existing U.S. global health platforms and programs.

*FIGURE 20: PROJECTED PREMATURE LUNG CANCER DEATHS IN U.S. PRIORITY COUNTRIES, 2014–2025*

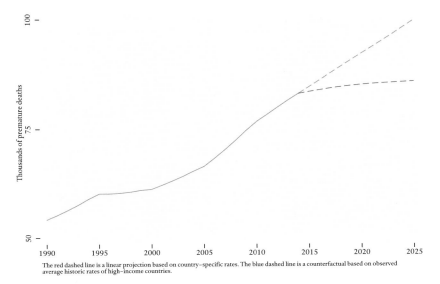

The red dashed line is a linear projection based on country-specific rates. The blue dashed line is a counterfactual based on observed average historic rates of high-income countries.

*Underlying Data Source:* Institute for Health Metrics and Evaluation, Global Burden of Disease Study 2013.

## POTENTIAL IMPACT

The potential benefits from increased U.S. leadership on international tobacco control are substantial. Deaths from tobacco generally occur years after its use. Nevertheless, as a rough and very partial indication of the potential benefits of U.S. leadership in tobacco, the Task Force has projected the expected increase in lung cancer deaths in the forty-nine U.S. priority countries by 2025 and the increase that would exist if those countries made improvements at the same rate that the average high-income country did between 2000 and 2013 (Figure 20). The difference between those projections just for lung cancer in these countries is 80,464 premature deaths and 135,831 deaths overall. Tobacco use and secondhand smoke are also leading risk factors for nearly all the NCDs identified by this Task Force as short- and near-term priorities.

## LIVER CANCER

The hepatitis B virus (HBV) is transmitted through bodily fluids and attacks the liver, causing chronic disease.[156] It is the source of most cases of liver cancer and each year is responsible for five hundred thousand deaths globally. In low- and middle-income countries, most hepatitis B transmission occurs early, from mother to infant.[157] The prevalence of this virus is greater and increasing in low- and middle-income countries, especially in sub-Saharan Africa and East Asia (Figure 21).

### AVAILABILITY OF PROVEN INTERVENTIONS

A safe and highly effective HBV vaccine is cheap and widely used.[158] The complete series of the HBV vaccine provides twenty years, and possibly lifelong, protection in infants, children, and young adults.[159] HBV vaccination is also the most effective means of reducing the risk of liver cancer from aflatoxin, a carcinogenic byproduct of fungi on grains and other crops common in tropical countries with poor food safety

*FIGURE 21: CHANGE IN PREMATURE LIVER CANCER DEATHS IN U.S. PRIORITY COUNTRIES, 1990–2013*

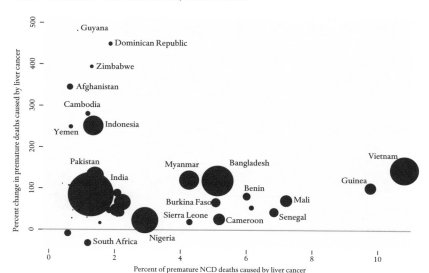

*Data Source:* Institute for Health Metrics and Evaluation, Global Burden of Disease Study 2013.

regimes.[160] A three-dose series of this vaccine costs less than two dollars through UNICEF and is eligible for subsidy by the GAVI Alliance. Although 179 of 193 WHO member states have introduced HBV vaccine into their immunization programs, coverage is suboptimal—an estimated 75 percent.[161] Many infants in sub-Saharan Africa and South Asia do not receive the first dose within twenty-four hours after birth, as needed.[162]

## WHAT THE UNITED STATES HAS TO OFFER

The countries in which children are not vaccinated for HBV are generally those with inadequate immunization programs. This Task Force recommends providing more technical and financial support for those child immunization programs; leveraging existing U.S. maternal and child health platforms to do so would help. This strategy may also yield compound benefits for controlling communicable diseases. Working with suppliers to package HBV vaccine in prefilled, auto-disable syringes appropriate for use in low-income countries would enable community-based health providers to deliver immunizations after home births, reducing the demand for health-care infrastructure in the poorest settings.[163]

## AVAILABLE COST ESTIMATES

Universal immunization with the HBV vaccine is cost-effective. Even at twice its current two-dollar price, the Disease Control Priority Network estimates that raising HBV immunization rates by another 25 percent would cost $122 million annually, save six hundred thousand lives annually, and generate a return on investment at a ratio of ten-to-one from reduced death and disability.[164] The Task Force's recommendation would cost considerably less but would help raise the priority of HBV vaccination in low-income countries and improve coverage rates.

## POTENTIAL IMPACT

Most vaccine-preventable diseases result in death at an early age, but deaths from liver cancer caused by hepatitis B happen years into the future. Countries that introduce hepatitis B vaccination today will experience significant benefits, but not for some time.[165] Ten years is

too short a period in which to exhibit the full health gains. Nevertheless, as a rough indication of the potential benefits of U.S. leadership
in the area, the Task Force has projected the expected increase in liver
cancer deaths in the forty-nine U.S. priority countries by 2025 and the
increase that would exist if those countries made improvements at the
same rate that the average high-income country did between 2000 and
2013 (Figure 22). The difference between those projections is 93,187 premature deaths and 230,090 deaths overall.

*FIGURE 22: PROJECTED PREMATURE LIVER CANCER DEATHS IN
U.S. PRIORITY COUNTRIES, 2014–2025*

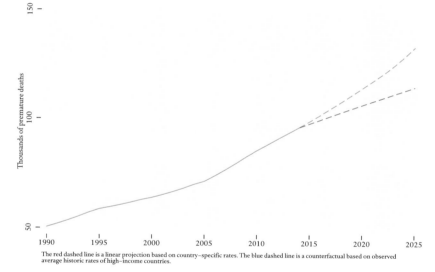

The red dashed line is a linear projection based on country–specific rates. The blue dashed line is a counterfactual based on observed average historic rates of high–income countries.

*Underlying Data Source:* Institute for Health Metrics and Evaluation, Global Burden of Disease Study 2013.

## CERVICAL CANCER

Approximately three hundred thousand women die from cervical
cancer each year, mostly young women in low- and middle-income
countries. Cervical cancer is now the leading cause of death from cancer
among women in sub-Saharan Africa and is a persistent, rising health
challenge in the developing countries where the United States has other
investments (Figure 23).

FIGURE 23: CHANGE IN PREMATURE CERVICAL CANCER DEATHS
IN U.S. PRIORITY COUNTRIES, 1990–2013

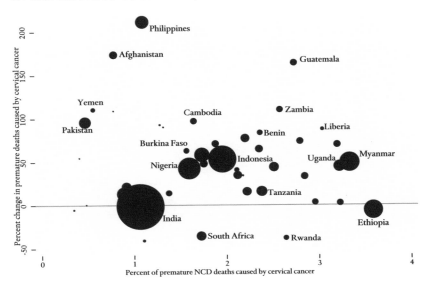

Data Source: Institute for Health Metrics and Evaluation, Global Burden of Disease Study 2013.

A century ago, cervical cancer was as common in the United States as it is today in low- and middle-income countries. Screening to identify cancerous lesions and advances in effective treatment produced a steep decline in cervical cancer incidence and mortality in the United States and other high-income countries.[166]

## AVAILABILITY OF PROVEN INTERVENTIONS

Most cervical cancer is caused by persistent infection with one of several strains of HPV. Two interventions could transform cervical cancer control in low- and middle-income countries: increased access to the effective vaccines that exist for preventing HPV infection; and implementation of screening methods that are more compatible with the available resources and infrastructure in developing countries than Pap smear programs.

Two HPV vaccines exist, and they are safe and highly effective in women aged thirteen to twenty-six. These vaccines require three doses over six months and have been proven to remain effective for at least five years when all doses are given, although the protective period may be longer.[167] The WHO has prequalified these vaccines, and they have also been approved for use by regulatory authorities in more than one hundred countries.

In 2012, the GAVI Alliance announced it would help support access to a sustainable supply of HPV vaccines at a price of $4.50 per dose in the poorest countries and fund demonstration programs. Countries introducing HPV vaccines must meet GAVI's co-financing requirement.[168] These same vaccines cost more than a hundred dollars per dose in high-income countries; the lowest reported public-sector price for developing countries that are not poor enough to qualify for GAVI support is thirteen dollars per dose.

A recent study found that most of the countries in which HPV vaccination would prevent the greatest number of cervical cancers are in sub-Saharan Africa, South Asia, and parts of Latin America, but that few have national HPV vaccination programs.[169] One exception is Rwanda, which reported vaccinating more than 93 percent of its adolescent girls against HPV in 2013—a spectacular achievement that proves HPV immunization can work in low-income settings.[170]

For women older than twenty-six, HPV vaccines cannot help. Cost-effective screening and treatment programs for precancerous lesions using direct visualization and cryotherapy—or, when those are not suitable, the loop electrosurgical excision procedure (LEEP)—have been piloted in low- and middle-income countries with good results.[171] Cervical screening should start when a woman is in her thirties and occur at least once or twice in her lifetime.[172]

## WHAT THE UNITED STATES HAS TO OFFER

Co-financing a national HPV vaccination program is a challenge for many low- and middle-income countries. Leaving aside the still-high price per dose, the vaccine must be delivered to a different age group than those who receive childhood immunizations and therefore requires development of new delivery programs. The nonprofit global health organization PATH has worked with low- and middle-income countries' governments to assess HPV vaccination and found that delivery costs average one to four dollars per dose.[173] These additional costs make the investment in HPV vaccination a difficult decision for these governments.

The United States should help by increasing assistance to low- and middle-income countries seeking to lower HPV vaccine delivery costs and improve efficiency. It should also evaluate the opportunities and feasibility of leveraging existing U.S. platforms in health, development, and education. These platforms could help reduce the barriers to introducing and scaling the rollout of the HPV vaccine.[174]

The Task Force recommends that the United States increase its investment in improving and integrating low-technology screen-and-treat programs for cervical cancer into PEPFAR platforms, building on the lessons of the successful Zambia pilot.[175] There are other good examples of cervical cancer screening programs using nurses or midwives in sub-Saharan Africa that the United States should evaluate.[176] The Pink Ribbon Red Ribbon initiative has been, and should continue to be, a good partner for the U.S. government in this area.

### AVAILABLE COST ESTIMATES

A recent comprehensive study rated HPV vaccination, under current cost assumptions, as "very cost-effective" in 87 percent of the 179 countries assessed under the standard metrics for medical interventions.[177] HPV vaccination was rated as "very cost-effective" in all but two of the forty-nine U.S. priority countries and as "cost-effective" in the others (Jordan and Yemen).[178] The WHO has developed a tool that countries and donors can use to estimate the costs of introducing the HPV vaccine to specific regions or nationally, the total cost per HPV vaccine dose, and the total cost per fully immunized girl.[179]

### POTENTIAL IMPACT

Cervical cancer is increasingly becoming a health threat experienced only by poor women in poor countries. With increased U.S. leadership, more may be done to help local governments address the needs of this underserved population. As with tobacco control and HBV vaccination, the returns of cervical cancer screening and vaccination are enormous but often only apparent in the long term. Nevertheless, as a very rough indication of the potential benefits of U.S. engagement, the Task Force has projected the expected increase in cervical cancer deaths in the forty-nine U.S. priority countries by 2025 and the increase that would exist if those countries improved at the same rate that the average high-income country did between 2000 and 2013 (Figure 24). The difference between those projections would be 48,865 premature deaths and 118,802 deaths overall.

FIGURE 24: PROJECTED PREMATURE CERVICAL CANCER DEATHS
IN U.S. PRIORITY COUNTRIES, 2014–2025

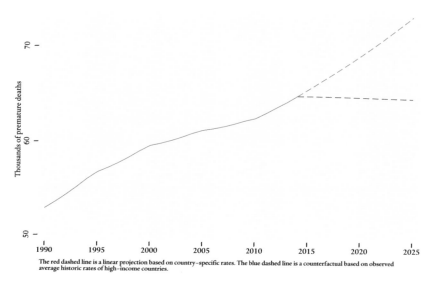

The red dashed line is a linear projection based on country-specific rates. The blue dashed line is a counterfactual based on observed average historic rates of high-income countries.

Underlying Data Source: Institute for Health Metrics and Evaluation, Global Burden of Disease Study 2013.

# NCD Challenges on Which
# U.S. Leadership Would Make a Difference
# in the Near Term

The Task Force has identified several NCD challenges for which effective interventions are widely used in the United States and other high-income countries but are not yet sufficiently low-cost or usable in low-infrastructure settings. Each challenge is especially prevalent among working-age populations in low- and middle-income countries where the United States has existing platforms that provide the opportunity for action. With U.S. leadership, more population and implementation research, and collaboration with private-sector and philanthropic partners, progress on adapting these interventions for cost-effective, low-infrastructure use is foreseeable in the near term.[180]

## TREATABLE AND CURABLE CANCERS

Tremendous progress has occurred in the United States and other high-income countries toward preventing and treating many cancers. Mammography screening, endocrine treatment, discovery of biomarkers, and systemic chemotherapy have reduced U.S. breast cancer death rates by one-third between 1990 and 2014, mostly in younger women.[181] A large proportion of cancers affecting children and young adults are now also highly curable in high-income countries, in particular leukemia and lymphomas, retinoblastoma, and testicular cancer.[182] Screening tests for *Helicobacter pylori*—a bacterium associated with stomach cancer—and treatment with antibiotics have helped cut stomach cancer death rates in high-income countries by 20 percent over twenty years.[183]

Although these cancers are treatable, curable, and declining in high-income countries, they are increasing and causing substantial suffering in poor countries. Between 1990 and 2013, premature deaths in low-income countries from breast cancer and leukemia grew 90 percent and 25 percent, respectively.[184] Similar patterns are seen in the countries where the United States has significant global health investments (Figures 25 and 26).

The reason for this disparity is that people in poor countries have little access to the diagnostic and curative care that is widely available for breast cancer and leukemia in wealthier countries. The per capita cost of mammography screening exceeds the capacity of many low-income countries to pay and may not be appropriate for settings wherein women often present with easily palpable, visible, or ulcerated tumors.[185] Appropriate breast cancer treatment depends on an accurate pathology diagnosis, which in turn requires the availability of tissue sampling procedures. Chemotherapy and radiotherapy are available on a limited basis in middle-income countries, but often not in poorer nations.

*FIGURE 25: CHANGE IN PREMATURE BREAST CANCER DEATHS IN U.S. PRIORITY COUNTRIES, 1990–2013*

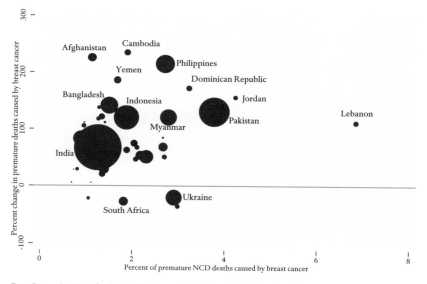

*Data Source:* Institute for Health Metrics and Evaluation, Global Burden of Disease Study 2013.

*FIGURE 26: CHANGE IN PREMATURE LEUKEMIA DEATHS IN U.S. PRIORITY COUNTRIES, 1990–2013*

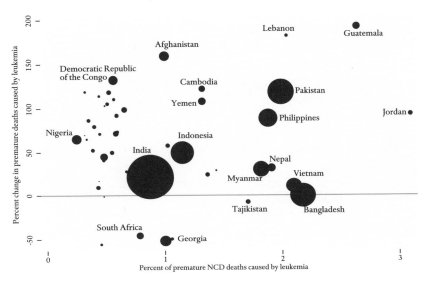

*Data Source:* Institute for Health Metrics and Evaluation, Global Burden of Disease Study 2013.

## POTENTIAL INTERVENTIONS

There are at least four ways that the United States may assist low- and lower-middle-income countries in addressing breast cancer, leukemia, and other treatable or curable cancers.

First, this Task Force recommends that the United States devote more resources to supporting registries in developing countries. Reliable, population-based registries define the incidence, mortality, and survival rates of different types of cancers and are fundamental to the development of local and national plans for improving cancer prevention and treatment.[186] The International Agency for Research on Cancer (IARC), the WHO, and others recently finalized standardized guidelines for the planning and development of population-based cancer registries in developing countries.[187] This is an important first step, but more is needed to support IARC in establishing regional hubs to provide training and technical assistance in setting up registries. NCI has important programs in these areas, but they are limited relative to the high demand.

Second, the Task Force calls on U.S. leadership to help mobilize support for development of resource-level-appropriate guidelines for the management of treatable and curable cancers. Breast cancer provides a good model. With the support of the Susan G. Komen Foundation and NCI, the Breast Health Global Initiative was formed and has since produced a comprehensive set of resource-specific, stage-specific guidelines for breast cancer management.[188] These guidelines provide the basis for prioritizing scarce local government resources and the blueprint for future investments. Similar guidelines are needed for leukemia and other treatable and curable cancers.

Third, the Task Force finds that more U.S. support is needed for research and NGOs such as PATH that are working to lower the costs and infrastructure demands of breast cancer screening and diagnosis. Examples of promising approaches are community-based breast cancer screening models and frugal diagnostic technologies, such as cheaper and easier-to-use core-needle devices.[189]

Fourth, the Task Force believes the United States should explore avenues for increasing "telepathology" programs between U.S. public hospitals and developing countries. These programs have been successfully used to build specialist capacity in Tanzania and Rwanda and create links with U.S. and European hospitals. More are needed.

Through these and other initiatives, the United States can help low- and middle-income countries build the foundation for addressing curable and treatable cancers. The greatest impact on mortality would come from earlier detection, more accurate diagnosis, and more widely available basic treatment. The potential benefits are significant. For example, the Task Force has estimated the current projected increase in premature death rates in the forty-nine U.S. priority countries by 2025 and the increase that would exist if those countries improved at the same rate that the average high-income country did between 2000 and 2013 (Figure 27). The difference is 110,617 premature deaths and 173,672 deaths overall.

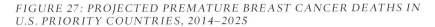

*FIGURE 27: PROJECTED PREMATURE BREAST CANCER DEATHS IN U.S. PRIORITY COUNTRIES, 2014–2025*

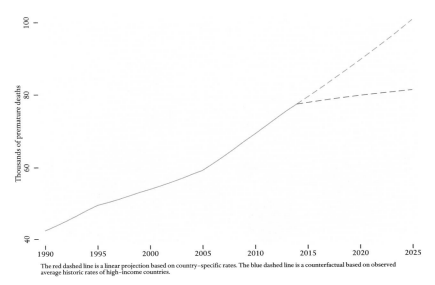

The red dashed line is a linear projection based on country–specific rates. The blue dashed line is a counterfactual based on observed average historic rates of high–income countries.

*Underlying Data Source:* Institute for Health Metrics and Evaluation, Global Burden of Disease Study 2013.

## DIABETES

Diabetes presents a special challenge in the Task Force's recommended strategy for stemming the rising tide of NCDs in low- and middle-income countries. On treatment, it offers a similar investment case as cardiovascular disease. There are also low-cost, long-off-patent medications for diabetes control. Metformin and insulin have existed since the1920s. Programs to monitor blood glucose levels and manage diabetes have been successfully integrated with HIV/AIDS and hypertension programs in Cambodia and can be piloted elsewhere.[190] Diabetes is a rising health challenge in the same countries where the United States has significant global health investments (Figure 28). Premature deaths from diabetes in these countries increased 82 percent between 1990 and 2013.

The challenge that diabetes presents is that, unlike with cardiovascular disease, the widespread availability of effective diabetes treatments and blood glucose monitoring has not sparked a dramatic decline in premature mortality in high-income countries. Under-age-sixty deaths

FIGURE 28: CHANGE IN PREMATURE DIABETES DEATHS IN U.S.
PRIORITY COUNTRIES, 1990–2013

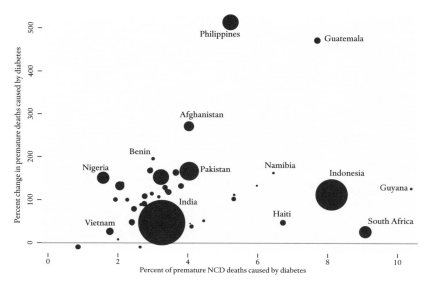

Data Source: Institute for Health Metrics and Evaluation, Global Burden of Disease Study 2013.

from diabetes increased 14 percent between 2000 and 2013 in high-income countries, which already had a high disease burden. The reason is the spectacular increases in the prevalence of the disease and its underlying risk factors—obesity, physical inactivity, excessive alcohol consumption, high salt intake, and others. Although the rates of these risk factors are lower in most developing countries, particularly relative to the United States, they are nonetheless increasing.

## POTENTIAL INTERVENTIONS

The Task Force recommends that the United States evaluate, pilot, and consider integrating diabetes objectives into hypertension procurement, management, and registries. There is also an important need to explore interventions on juvenile diabetes. Deaths from this disease are rare in high-income countries, but are believed to be high in low-income countries where treatment and blood glucose monitoring programs are unavailable. These strategies have the potential to slow the increasing rate of premature mortality from diabetes and save a significant number of lives (Figure 29).

*FIGURE 29: PROJECTED PREMATURE DIABETES DEATHS IN U.S.*
*PRIORITY COUNTRIES, 2014–2025*

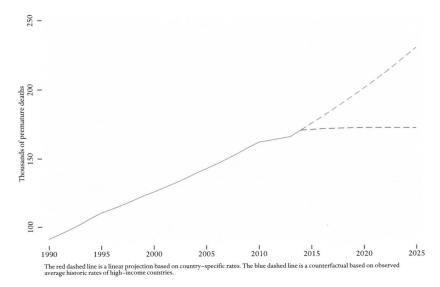

The red dashed line is a linear projection based on country–specific rates. The blue dashed line is a counterfactual based on observed average historic rates of high–income countries.

*Underlying Data Source:* Institute for Health Metrics and Evaluation, Global Burden of Disease Study 2013.

Over the long term, it will be difficult to make progress in reducing the premature deaths and disability from diabetes without more effective population-based prevention and nutrition programs. These are challenges that the United States shares and are some of the topics discussed in the final section of this report.

# Shared NCD Challenges
for Collaboration

There are many NCD challenges for which no effective interventions yet exist in developed or developing countries. These are the areas wherein closer collaboration between the United States, developing countries, and private-sector partners would have the greatest benefits.

## DEVELOPING- AND EMERGING-COUNTRY PARTNERS

There is no long-term treatment solution to the challenge of NCDs. Only prevention can reduce the burden of these diseases and lower their associated health-care costs to sustainable levels. This is true for the United States, but particularly so for developing countries with limited resources. The targets of NCD prevention are well known: salt intake, obesity, physical inactivity, excessive alcohol consumption, poor nutrition, consumption of trans fats, and indoor air pollution. The strategies for addressing those challenges are less established, at least not in a manner that can be applied cost-effectively, at the population level, and across different settings.

The United States and developing countries may have much to learn from each other on prevention. The United States may finally be making progress on its enormous childhood obesity problem, although that remains hotly debated.[191] If it is, however, it would be the first (albeit tentative) sign of an effective anti-obesity campaign. Few population-based campaigns to increase physical activity have succeeded, but Brazil and Colombia have conducted initiatives that achieved positive results.[192]

Nutrition is another promising area for collaboration between developed and developing countries on prevention. Many vegetables and fruits are disappearing from diets globally. More and more people are subsisting on fewer and fewer crops.[193] Inadequate access to fruits and vegetables is associated with diabetes, heart disease, and certain cancers and results in a surprisingly high number of deaths around the world (2.7 million annually).[194] Low- and middle-income countries are leading initiatives, in some cases with U.S. funding, to incentivize smallholder farm production, promote urban gardens, and integrate nutrition and healthy diet promotion into primary care.[195] If successful, the approaches pioneered in countries such as Ethiopia and Honduras might also have relevance in the United States and other high-income countries.[196]

As far as treatment is concerned, developing countries lead the way in experimenting with lower-cost chronic care models. Identification and scale-up of affordable NCD prevention and treatments of NCDs in these settings may help slow the spectacular rise of health costs in the United States and other developed countries.[197] One area of particular need is mental health.[198] Without an adequate mental health–care component, initiatives to address NCDs are more costly and less effective.[199] The WHO estimates that nearly two hundred million people worldwide suffer from depression or schizophrenia, making the conditions a leading cause of disability globally.[200] Sufferers of mental illness are twice as likely to smoke cigarettes, more apt to be obese, and more likely to have multiple NCDs.[201] Individuals with three or more NCDs generate more than 80 percent of U.S. Medicare costs.[202]

Effective and affordable models of mental health care exist. Randomized clinical trials in the United States have shown that integrating treatment into primary care improves the quality and outcomes of that care.[203] Ethiopia, India, Nepal, South Africa, and Uganda have piloted basic mental health treatment packages, including offering access via their primary-care platforms to some or all of the medications on the WHO essential drug list.[204] More research is needed to examine how to best train health workers, reduce stigma, and build public support for effective implementation of such programs in low-resource settings in developed and developing countries.

This Task Force recommends that the United States propose adding NCD prevention, diagnosis, and treatment to the agendas of its regular bilateral dialogues with Brazil, China, India, and Indonesia.[205] These dialogues occur annually and provide a framework for building trust, constructive engagement, and collaboration on issues of shared strategic and economic interest. Past agendas for these dialogues have included clean energy and promoting scientific collaboration.[206] The premature and preventable burden of NCDs is enormous in these emerging nations, and an important issue for collaboration with the United States.

## PRIVATE-SECTOR PARTNERS

The role for the business community in addressing NCDs in low- and middle-income countries is threefold. First, many companies have natural concerns about maintaining the health and productivity of their workforces and the size and purchasing power of their customer bases. A 2010 World Economic Forum survey revealed that executives operating in South Asia and low-income countries had expressed the greatest concerns about the rise of NCDs.[207] Many of these executives' companies are leading the way in designing and implementing innovative health promotion programs for their employees that emphasize exercise, preventive care, better diets, and reduced smoking. These programs may prove transferrable to broader populations.

Second, voluntary programs and partnerships with food and beverage suppliers and retailers will be critical for progress on a number of NCD risk factors. Many developing-country governments lack the capacity and popular support for implementing tax and regulatory measures to change diets. The UK Food Standards Agency reduced salt intake by 15 percent, primarily through voluntary agreements with manufacturers to reformulate products.[208] Such agreements are proving far more effective than attempts to inspire population-level behavior change in individual cooking and eating habits.[209] More voluntary and independently audited agreements are needed to lower salt intake in other countries as well as to reduce trans fats, unhealthy oils, sugars, and the marketing of unhealthy food and beverages to children. These negotiations should be coordinated by regional health authorities, be facilitated by the U.S. development agencies, and involve leaders from the public health community and manufacturers and retailers.

Third, the private sector is best suited to invent and adapt technologies for NCD prevention and treatment in low-infrastructure settings. Pharmaceutical, medical device, and information technology companies can develop and distribute effective and affordable diagnostics, therapies, and information systems needed to lower NCD prevention, detection, and treatment costs. Frugal technologies developed for low-income settings may prove popular for high-income-country use. General Electric (GE) has made this approach, known as reverse innovation, a core part of its health-care business model.[210] GE developed a portable electrocardiographic diagnostic tool for India that costs one-fifth of the price of the high-income-country model. This portable electrocardiogram is now reportedly popular among German primary-care physicians.[211]

The Task Force has identified three areas in which further innovation and private-sector participation are needed: clean cookstoves, breast cancer diagnostics, and the use of information and communication technologies (eHealth) and mobile phones (mHealth) to support NCD prevention and management.

Indoor air pollution is among the top five health risks for developing countries and a particular challenge for women who do most of the meal preparation in these settings. The WHO estimates that three billion people cook and heat their homes using open fires and simple stoves, burning biomass (wood, animal dung, and crop waste) and coal.[212] The Global Alliance for Clean Cookstoves is doing good work, but generating cleaner, low-cost stoves that respond to local needs, tastes, and customs is difficult. More private-sector engagement and innovative partnerships with developing country entrepreneurs might help.

Mammography screening is still too expensive and resource-intensive for widespread use in many developing countries to address rising breast cancer rates. Clinical breast examinations might help if cheaper diagnostic technologies were available that could be used by nurses and other lower-skilled health workers. With radiotherapy and chemotherapy unavailable in many low- and middle-income countries, mastectomies would remain the best treatment option, but they are only effective with early and accurate diagnosis.[213]

Despite the intuitive appeal of cell phones as a low-cost way to reach large numbers of people in low-infrastructure settings, the early results of eHealth and mHealth initiatives are not encouraging.[214] Further innovation is needed, and the private sector is likely to be best suited to succeed in this area.

This Task Force recommends that the U.S. government act as a convener of multinational corporations and NGOs working to apply and adapt cost-effective technology for NCDs in low-infrastructure developing-country settings. The purpose would be to coordinate and scale private-sector creativity and assets around critical NCD-related needs for which the market potential is not yet realized. The White House, Department of State, and USAID have hosted similar efforts on global health and international development, but those meetings did not address NCDs or their risk factors.[215] USAID should also incorporate NCDs into its Grand Challenges program, which leverages outside funding to support research on U.S. development priorities, and the Development Innovation Ventures fund, which provides seed capital to high-risk, high-return, development-friendly technologies.[216]

# Conclusion

Global health is in transition. The exotic parasites, bacterial blights, and communicable diseases that have long occupied international health initiatives remain important but are declining in most countries. That is good news, but this epidemiological transition is not yielding the demographic and economic benefits that accompanied that transition in wealthier countries. Cancers, heart disease, and other NCDs are increasing in prevalence faster, arising in younger populations, and having worse outcomes than in wealthy nations. Unless urgent action is taken, this emerging global health crisis will worsen and become harder to address.

Just as low- and middle-income governments must adapt and retool to confront their changing health demands, so too must the United States and other international actors that have invested in global health. It is not sustainable to continue to invest billions fighting treatable and preventable diseases only to watch the same patients perish prematurely as a result of equally treatable and preventable conditions, and in increasing numbers. This is especially true for those NCDs for which many premature deaths are avoidable with relatively low cost.

U.S. interests in addressing HIV/AIDS, malaria, and poor reproductive and maternal health lay not in these diseases and conditions themselves, but in the well-being and fortunes of the countries and working-age people that suffer from them. The same interests exist with NCDs. As the scale and consequence of this NCD epidemic grows rapidly in low- and middle-income countries, so will the threat to U.S. interests.

This Task Force is under no illusion that the recommendations and strategies outlined in this report are alone sufficient to stem the tide of NCDs in developing countries. Building health systems, allocating scarce resources, and enforcing public health laws and consumer protections are decisions for national governments alone. Yet the priorities of the United States and global health actors deeply influence those decisions. The recommendations and strategies outlined in this report would save lives, demonstrate the feasibility of progress on NCDs, and catalyze broader action. The time to act is now.

This Task Force recommends two immediate steps. First, the U.S. government must undertake a serious examination of its current global health priorities and spending and act to ensure their continued effectiveness in advancing U.S. interests. That examination should consider the potential for additional funds and the feasibility of expanding the mandate of U.S. programs from disease-focused objectives to more outcome-oriented measures for improving the health of the populations targeted.

Second, the United States should convene the leading actors and potential partners on addressing NCDs—national governments; intergovernmental and international institutions such as the WHO, World Bank, Global Fund, and GAVI Alliance; philanthropic foundations and NGOs; and private companies, especially large-scale employers operating in low- and middle-income countries. If the United States devoted resources to addressing NCDs in similar amounts as it spends on other global health priorities ($236 million on TB in FY 2014), it would go a long way toward implementing the recommendations outlined in this report.[217] Those costs, however, should not be borne by the United States alone. The purpose of this convening should be to develop a practical, well-prioritized, and sustainable plan for collective action on the emerging global health crisis of NCDs in low- and middle-income countries.

# Additional Views

The Task Force report does an excellent job outlining the challenges and some of the strategies dealing with noncommunicable diseases in the developing world, and for that reason I endorse it.

But the report does not fully include diet, nutrition, and other forms of preventative care as key strategies to help stem the tide of diabetes, cardiac problems, hypertension, cancers, and other medical conditions. The report does mention that nutrition is a promising area for collaboration between developed and developing countries on prevention. Inadequate access to fruits and vegetables is associated with diabetes, heart disease, and certain cancers and results in a surprising high number of deaths around the world. And the report does indicate that "dietary factors" are the single leading health risk in developing countries. Yet the report gives short shrift to identifying public-health solutions and strategies that directly address these dietary factors and nutritional deficiencies, especially in ensuring balanced diets in the developing world. In recent years, many organizations, including the UN's World Food Programme, the U.S. Agency for International Development, the U.S. Departments of Agriculture and Health and Human Services, as well as various NGOs, foundations, and private sector companies have all identified poor nutrition as a leading factor in child stunting and other diseases, including adult-onset diabetes and cancer. The evidence is legion that poor nutrition and an unbalanced diet are major contributors to these diseases, and good diets have a particularly important role in buttressing immune systems. In the same way that the report underscores the importance of reducing tobacco consumption, hypertension, and cancer rates, as well as increasing access to modern medicines, we also need to highlight strategies that better integrate food and nutrition, as well as improved food and water safety, into our more traditional clinical strategies, and consider them a key part of the total picture.

The basic health-care infrastructure of the developing world needs holistic solutions to deal with these noncommunicable diseases, which include the strategies contained in the report, modern medicine, good sanitation, and adequate and balanced food intake. Modern medicine has been outstanding in working on cures for diseases, but in my judgment the medical community has not given the same attention to prevention as a way to deal with disease. That includes diet and nutrition. As the French author Anthelme Brillat-Savarin wrote nearly two hundred years ago, "Tell me what you eat, and I will tell you what you are." Or in more colloquial terms, you are what you eat. A huge part of our effort to prevent disease and extend life should be rooted in that historical quotation.

Daniel R. Glickman

The Task Force report provides an important perspective and call to action to address NCDs in the most hard-hit and at-risk countries around the globe. The report accurately and rightfully acknowledges the critical toll NCDs are taking on political, social, and health systems in many countries. The challenges to preventing and treating NCDs are exacerbated in many of these countries because of under-resourced and underfunded health systems. Innovative and proactive programs must be implemented in the immediate term to help surmount the growing morbidity and mortality from NCDs in resource-limited settings.

The report articulates the perspective of U.S. interests and thus the incentives to help lead efforts to tackle this disease burden. Understandably, it is important to provide compelling reasons and to galvanize U.S. policymakers and spending authority to invest in the effort against NCDs; it is required to mobilize the needed support from the United States, a leader in global health. However, I would stress that the solutions—the actual programs, the policies, and final spending allocations towards particular NCDs—be done in close consultation and following the lead of host national governments. This approach will help ensure local buy-in and participation in solutions, which will increase their likelihood to succeed. For example, the report cites the success of Rwanda's HPV vaccination program. This success is in large part because it was a national priority instigated by the ministry and thus implemented in an embraceable and scalable manner. This country-led approach often requires patience and flexibility, but it is also often more efficient and effective in the long run.[218]

Vanessa Kerry

# Endnotes

1.  The figures and tables in this report fall into three categories and are sourced accordingly. Figures and tables that are original to this report and based on data that does not appear elsewhere but that have been generated using data from another source indicate their "underlying data source." Figures and tables that are original to this report but produced with data from another source indicate their "data source." Figures and tables that appear elsewhere and are not original to this report indicate their "source."

2.  Lisa A. Lee et al., "The Estimated Mortality Impact of Vaccinations Forecast to be Administered During 2011–2020 in 73 Countries Supported by the GAVI Alliance," *Vaccine* vol. 31 (2013), pp. B61–B72, doi: 10.1016/j.vaccine.2012.11.035; Eran Bendavid and Jayanta Bhattacharya, "The President's Emergency Plan for AIDS Relief in Africa: An Evaluation of Outcomes," *Annals of Internal Medicine* vol. 150 (2009), pp. 688–95, doi:10.7326/0003-4819-150-10-200905190-00117.

3.  The World Bank categorizes countries by the gross national income (GNI) per capita. There are thirty-four low-income countries, defined as those nations with a GNI per capita of $1,045 or less in 2013. There are fifty lower-middle-income countries, which are those with a GNI per capita of $4,125 or less in the same year. There are fifty-five high-middle-income countries, which had a GNI per capita of not more than $12,746 in 2013. See World Bank Data, "Country and Lending Groups," http://data.worldbank.org/about/country-and-lending-groups. This report uses the terms "developing countries" and "low- and middle-income countries" interchangeably. A list of the countries in these income groups can be found in the online Annex to this report, available at www.cfr.org/NCDs_Task_Force.

4.  David Stuckler, "Population Causes and Consequences of Leading Chronic Diseases: A Comparative Analysis of Prevailing Explanations," *Milbank Quarterly* vol. 86 (2008), pp. 273–326, doi: 10.1111/j.1468-0009.2008.00522.x.

5.  World Health Organization (WHO), "Global Status Report on Non-Communicable Diseases 2010," April 2011, http://whqlibdoc.who.int/publications/2011/9789240686458_eng.pdf?ua=1, p. 10.

6.  "The Good News About Cancer in Developing Countries," *Lancet* vol. 378 (2011), p. 1605, doi: 10.1016/S0140-6736(11)61681-4.

7.  WHO, "Global Status Report on Non-Communicable Diseases 2010," p. 9.

8.  Dean T. Jamison et al., "Global Health 2035: A World Converging Within a Generation," *Lancet* vol. 382 (2013), pp. 1898–955, doi: 10.1016/S0140-6736(13)62105-4.

9.  Alexandra Cameron et al., "Differences in the Availability of Medicines for Chronic and Acute Conditions in the Public and Private Sectors of Developing Countries," *Bulletin of the World Health Organization* vol. 89 (2011), pp. 412–21, doi: 10.2471/BLT.10.084327.

10. WHO, "Global Status Report on Non-Communicable Diseases 2010," p. 37.

11. Hacinthe Tchewonpi Kankeu et al., "The Financial Burden From Non-Communicable Diseases in Low- and Middle-Income Countries: A Literature Review," *Health Research Policy and Systems* vol. 11 (2013), doi: 10.1186/1478-4505-11-31.

12. Hind Elrayah et al., "Economic Burden on Families of Childhood Type 1 Diabetes in Urban Sudan," *Diabetes Research and Clinical Practice* vol. 70 (2005), pp. 159–165.

13. Ama de-Graft Aikins, "Healer Shopping in Africa: New Evidence From Rural–Urban Qualitative Study of Ghanaian Diabetes Experiences," *BMJ* vol. 331 (2005), doi:http://dx.doi.org/10.1136/bmj.331.7519.737.

14. Michael M. Engelgau et al., "Capitalizing on the Demographic Transition: Tackling Noncommunicable Diseases in South Asia," World Bank, June 2011, http://elibrary.worldbank.org/doi/pdf/10.1596/978-0-8213-8724-5.

15. Valentín Fuster and Bridget B. Kelly, eds., *Promoting Cardiovascular Health in the Developing World: A Critical Challenge to Achieve Global Health* (Washington, DC: The National Academies Press, 2010), pp. 136–43; Robert Beaglehole et al., "UN High Level Meeting on Non-Communicable Diseases: Addressing Four Questions," *Lancet* vol. 378 (2011), p. 450, doi: 10.1016/S0140-6736(11)60879-9.

16. David Bloom et al., "The Global Economic Burden of Non-Communicable Diseases," World Economic Forum, September 2011, p. 11, http://www3.weforum.org/docs/WEF_Harvard_HE_GlobalEconomicBurdenNonCommunicableDiseases_2011.pdf; Hendrina A. de Boo and Jane E. Harding, "The Developmental Origin of Adult Disease (Barker) Hypothesis," *Australian and New Zealand Journal of Obstetrics and Gynaecology* vol. 46 (2006), pp. 4–14, doi: 10.1111/j.1479-828X.2006.00506.x.

17. Irina A. Nikolic, Anderson E. Stanciole, and Mikhail Zaydman, "Chronic Emergency: Why NCDs Matter," World Bank Health, Nutrition, and Population Discussion Paper, July 2011, pp. 6, 9–10, http://siteresources.worldbank.org/HEALTHNUTRITIONANDPOPULATION/Resources/281627-1095698140167/ChronicEmergencyWhyNCDsMatter.pdf.

18. Nikolic, Stanciole, and Zaydman, "Chronic Emergency," p. 6; Engelgau et al., "Capitalizing on the Demographic Transition," p. 21.

19. Paulo Prada, "Special Report: Why Brazil's New Middle Class is Seething," Reuters, July 4, 2013, http://www.reuters.com/article/2013/07/03/us-brazil-middle-specialreport-idUSBRE9620DT20130703.

20. Bloom et al., "The Global Economic Burden of Non-Communicable Diseases," p. 29; Dele O. Abegunde et al., "The Burden and Costs of Chronic Diseases in Low-Income and Middle-Income Countries," *Lancet* vol. 370 (2007), pp. 1929–38, doi: 10.1016/S0140-6736(07)61696-1.

21. Nikolic, Stanciole, and Zaydman, "Chronic Emergency."

22. Bloom et al., "The Global Economic Burden of Non-Communicable Diseases," p. 29; World Bank Data, "By Income Level," 2013, http://data.worldbank.org.

23. Charles Kenny, *Getting Better, Why Global Development is Succeeding* (New York: Basic Books, 2011), pp. 122, 125–6.

24. World Development Indicator Tables, "Life Expectancy at Birth (Total Years)," World Bank, http://data.worldbank.org/indicator/SP.DYN.LE00.IN.

25. Engelgau et al., "Capitalizing on the Demographic Transition," p. 3.

26. Daniel D. Reidpath and Pascale Allotey, "The Burden is Great and the Money Little: Changing Chronic Disease Management in Low- and Middle-Income Countries," *Journal of Global Health* vol. 2 (2012), doi: 10.7189/jogh.02.020301.

27. PriceWaterhouseCoopers, "From Vision to Decision: Pharma 2020," November 2012, http://download.pwc.com/ie/pubs/2012_pharma_2020.pdf.

28. Institute for Health Metrics and Evaluation, "Financing Global Health 2013: Transition in an Age of Austerity," 2014, pp. 61–62, http://www.healthdata.org/policy-report/ financing-global-health-2013-transition-age-austerity.

29. OECD (Organization for Economic Cooperation and Development) Health Stats, "Public Health Expenditure Since 2000," via Organization for Economic Cooperation and Development, http://stats.oecd.org/index.aspx?DataSetCode=HEALTH_STAT.

30. OECD Health Stats, "Public Health Expenditure Since 2000"; World Development Indicator Tables, "Population (Total)," via World Bank Data, http://data.worldbank. org/indicator/SP.POP.TOTL.

31. Thomas Reardon, C. Peter Timmer, and Bart Minten, "The Supermarket Revolution in Asia and Emerging Development Strategies to Include Small Farmers," *Proceedings of the National Academy of Science of the USA* vol. 109 (2010), pp. 12332–7, doi: 10.1073/ pnas.1003160108; Barry M. Popkin, Linda S Adair, and Shu Wen Ng, "Now and Then: The Global Nutrition Transition: The Pandemic of Obesity in Developing Countries," *Nutrition Reviews* vol. 70 (2011), pp. 3–21, doi: 10.1111/j.1753-4887.2011.00456.x; David Weatherspoon and Thomas Reardon, "The Rise of Supermarkets in Africa: Implications for Agrifood Systems and the Rural Poor," *Development Policy Review* vol. 21 (2003), pp. 333–35, doi:10.1111/1467-7679.00214.

32. Colin K. Khoury et al., "Increasing Homogeneity in Global Food Supplies and the Implications for Food Security," *PNAS* vol. 111 (2014), pp. 4001–6, doi: 10.1073/ pnas.1313490111.

33. Katharine M. Esson and Stephen R. Leeder, *The Millennium Development Goals and Tobacco Control* (Geneva: World Health Organization, 2004), p. xi.

34. Thomas J. Bollyky, "Developing Symptoms: Noncommunicable Diseases Go Global," *Foreign Affairs* vol. 91 (2012), pp. 136–37.

35. See, for example, Duff Wilson, "Tobacco Funds Shrink as Obesity Fight Intensifies," *New York Times*, July 2010, http://www.nytimes.com/2010/07/28/health/ policy/28obesity.html; Thomas J. Bollyky, "Beyond Ratification: The Future of U.S. Engagement on International Tobacco Control," Center for Strategic & International Studies, November 2010, pp. 12–13, http://csis.org/files/publication/111210_Bollyky_ ByndRatifica_WEB.pdf.

36. "Tobacco Company Files Claim Against Uruguay Over Labeling Laws," *Bridges* vol. 14, International Centre for Trade and Sustainable Development (2010), http://ictsd. org/i/news/bridgesweekly/71988/; Sabrina Tavernise, "Tobacco Firms' Strategy Limits Poorer Nations' Smoking Laws," *New York Times*, December 2013; Thomas J. Bollyky, "The Tobacco Problem in U.S. Trade," Council on Foreign Relations Press, September 2013.

37. Steven Allender et al., "Quantifying Urbanization as a Risk Factor for Noncommunicable Disease," *Journal of Urban Health* vol. 88 (2001), p. 906, doi: 10.1007/ s11524-011-9586-1.

38. United Nations (UN), "World Urbanization Prospects, 2014 Revision Highlights," pp. 13–15, http://esa.un.org/unpd/wup/Highlights/WUP2014-Highlights.pdf.

39. Tim Campbell and Alana Campbell, "Emerging Disease Burdens and the Poor in Cities of the Developing World," *Journal of Urban Health* vol. 84 (2007), p. i55, doi: 10.1007/s11524-007-9181-7.

40. UN, "World Economic and Social Survey: Sustainable Development Challenges" pp. 58–60, http://sustainabledevelopment.un.org/content/documents/2843WESS2013. pdf; Julie E. Fischer and Rebecca Katz, "The International Flow of Risk: The Governance of Health in an Urbanizing World," *Global Health Governance* vol. 4 (2011); Campbell et al., "Emerging Disease Burdens," p. i59.

41. Fischer et al., "International Flow of Risk," p. 4.

42. Barry M. Popkin, "Technology, Transport, Globalization, and Nutrition Transition Food Policy," *Food Policy* vol. 31 (2006), pp. 554–69, doi:10.1016/j.foodpol.2006.02.008.

43. Engelgau et al., "Capitalizing on the Demographic Transition"; David Stuckler, "Population Causes and Consequences of Leading Chronic Diseases: A Comparative Analysis of Prevailing Explanations," *Milbank Quarterly* vol. 86 (2008), pp. 273–326, doi: 10.1111/j.1468-0009.2008.00522.x.

44. See Annex, available at www.cfr.org/NCDs_Task_Force.

45. See Annex, available at www.cfr.org/NCDs_Task_Force.; Vivien Davis Tsu, Jose Jeronimo, and Benjamin O. Anderson, "Why the Time is Right to Tackle Breast and Cervical Cancer in Low-Resource Settings," *Bulletin of the World Health Organization* vol. 91 (2013), pp. 683–90, doi: http://dx.doi.org/10.2471/BLT.12.116020.

46. See Annex, available at www.cfr.org/NCDs_Task_Force.

47. Michael R. Reich and Priya Bery, "Expanding Global Access to ARVs: The Challenges of Prices and Patents" in Kenneth H. Mayer and H.F. Pizer, eds., *The AIDS Pandemic: Impact on Science and Society* (New York: New York Academic Press, 2005), p. 332.

48. Henry J. Kaiser Family Foundation, "The U.S. President's Emergency Plan for AIDS Relief (PEPFAR)," June 2014; PEPFAR Stewardship and Oversight Act of 2013, 113th Congress, Public Law No. 113-56, December 2, 2013.

49. Adapted from Adam Wexler and Jennifer Kates, "The U.S. Global Health Budget: Analysis of the Fiscal Year 2015 Budget Request," Henry J. Kaiser Family Foundation, March 2014, http://kff.org/global-health-policy/issue-brief/the-u-s-global-health-budget-analysis-of-the-fiscal-year-2015-budget-request.

50. Henry J. Kaiser Family Foundation, "The U.S. Government and Global Non-Communicable Diseases," April 2014.

51. Centers for Disease Control and Prevention (CDC), Office of the Director, "CDC Global Health Strategy 2012–15," June 2012, http://www.cdc.gov/globalhealth/strategy/pdf/CDC-GlobalHealthStrategy.pdf.

52. CDC Center for Global Health, "The Global Standardized Hypertension Treatment Project," http://www.cdc.gov/globalhealth/ncd/hypertension-treatment.htm.

53. U.S. Department of State, "Pink Ribbon Red Ribbon Overview," September 2011, http://www.state.gov/r/pa/prs/ps/2011/09/172244.htm.

54. Pink Ribbon Red Ribbon, "Annual Report 2013," http://pinkribbonredribbon.org/wp-content/uploads/pink-ribbon-red-ribbon-2013-annual-report.pdf.

55. Global Alliance for Clean Cookstoves, "The Cookstove Story," http://www.cleancookstoves.org.

56. U.S. Department of State, Office of the Spokesperson, "The United States' Commitment to the Global Alliance for Clean Cookstoves: Year Three Progress Report," September 2013, http://www.state.gov/r/pa/prs/ps/2013/09/214799.htm.

57. UCL Institute for Global Health, "Global Alliance for Chronic Diseases: An Alliance of Health Research Funders," http://www.gacd.org/about.

58. National Cancer Institute at the U.S. National Institutes of Health, "NCI Center for Global Health: Research Programs and Initaitives," http://www.cancer.gov/aboutnci/organization/global-health/research-programs-initiatives.

59. Fogarty International Center, "Chronic, Non-Communicable Diseases and Disorders Across the Lifespan: Fogarty International Research Training Award (NCD-LIFESPAN)," U.S. National Institutes of Health, http://www.fic.nih.gov/Programs/Pages/chronic-lifespan.aspx.

60. U.S. Agency for International Development (USAID), "Conceptual Framework on Noncommunicable Diseases and Injuries (NCDIs), Accelerating Progress on USAID's Existing Health Priorities," consultation draft.

61. Henry J. Kaiser Family Foundation, "The U.S. Government and Global Non-Communicable Diseases," April 2014, http://kff.org/global-health-policy/fact-sheet/the-u-s-government-and-global-non-communicable-diseases.

62. Institute for Health Metrics and Evaluation, "Financing Global Health 2013: Transition in an Age of Austerity."

63. WHO, "Global Burden of Disease Report," 1996, pp. 1, 14, 16–17.

64. WHO, "Global Action Plan for the Prevention and Control of Noncommunicable Diseases 2013–2020," 2013; Ruth Bonita et al., "Country Actions to Meet UN Commitments on Non-Communicable Diseases: A Stepwise Approach" *Lancet* vol. 381 (2013), doi: 10.1016/S0140-6736(12)61993-X.

65. WHO, "Universal Health Coverage: Report by the Secretariat," 132nd Session of the Executive Board, January 2013, http://apps.who.int/gb/ebwha/pdf_files/EB132/B132_22-en.pdf.

66. WHO, "Proposed Program Budget 2014–2015," 66th World Health Assembly, April 2013, http://www.who.int/about/resources_planning/A66_7-en.pdf?ua=1.

67. Institute for Health Metrics and Evaluation, "Financing Global Health 2013"; WHO, "Assessing National Capacity for the Prevention and Control of Noncommunicable Diseases: Report of the 2010 Global Survey," 2012.

68. Countries that were ineligible for DAH based on their World Bank income classification are shown in white. DAH received is shown in real 2011 U.S. dollars.

69. U.S. Office of Management and Budget, Agency Congressional Budget Justifications, Congressional Appropriation Bills and U.S. Foreign Assistance Dashboard, http://www.foreignassistance.gov.

70. WorldPublicOpinion.org, "International Public Opinion on Development and Aid," http://www.worldpublicopinion.org/pipa/articles/btdevelopmentaidra/index.php?nid=&id=&lb=btda.

71. Christopher J. L. Murray et al., "Global, Regional, and National Incidence and Mortality for HIV, Tuberculosis, and Malaria During 1990–2013: A Systematic Analysis for the Global Burden of Disease Study 2013," *Lancet* (2014), doi: 10.1016/S0140-6736(14)60844-8.

72. Lisa R. Hirschhorn et al., "Cancer and the 'Other' Noncommunicable Chronic Diseases in Older People Living With HIV/AIDS in Resource-Limited Settings: A Challenge to Success," *AIDS* vol. 26 (2012), pp. S65–S75.

73. Ibid, pp. 103–4.

74. International Union Against Tuberculosis and Lung Disease and World Health Organization, *Collaborative Framework for Care and Control of Tuberculosis and Diabetes* (Geneva: World Health Organization, 2011), whqlibdoc.who.int/publications/2011/9789241502252_eng.pdf.

75. Jo Leonardi-Bee, John Britton, and Andrea Venn, "Secondhand Smoke and Adverse Fetal Outcomes in Nonsmoking Pregnant Women: A Meta-Analysis," *Pediatrics* vol. 127 (2001), pp. 734–41, doi: 10.1542/peds.2010-3041; Giselle Salmasi et al., "Environmental Tobacco Smoke Exposure and Perinatal Outcomes: A Systematic Review and Meta-Analyses," *Acta Obstetricia et Gynecologica Scandinavica* vol. 89 (2010), pp. 23–41, doi: 10.3109/00016340903505748.

76. Stacey L. Knobler et al., eds., *The Infectious Etiology of Chronic Diseases: Defining the Relationship, Enhancing the Research, and Mitigating the Effects* (Washington, DC: National Academies Press, 2004).

77. Henry J. Kaiser Family Foundation, "U.S. Global Health Assistance, FY2013 by Program Area," 2014.

78. This analysis does not include South Sudan, which received more than $5 million in U.S. global health assistance, but for which IHME did not have data at time of publication; John Donnelly, "GHI Expands Focus Countries to 29," *Global Post*, November 2011, http://www.globalpost.com/dispatches/globalpost-blogs/global-pulse/ghi-expands-focus-countries-29.

79. USAID, "U.S. Foreign Assistance Dashboard," http://www.foreignassistance.gov/web/DataView.aspx.

80. See Annex, available at www.cfr.org/NCDs_Task_Force.

81. USAID, "Accelerating Progress on USAID's Existing Health Priorities."

82. International Diabetes Federation, *IDF Diabetes Atlas, Sixth Edition* (International Diabetes Federation, 2013), http://www.idf.org/sites/default/files/EN_6E_Atlas_Full_0.pdf.

83. Rafael Lozano et al., "Global and Regional Mortality From 235 Causes of Death for 20 Age Groups in 1990 and 2010: A Systematic Analysis for the Global Burden of Disease Study 2010," *Lancet* vol. 380 (2012), doi: 10.1016/S0140-6736(12)61728-0; Eloi Marijon et al., "Rheumatic Heart Disease," *Lancet* vol. 379 (2012), pp. 953–64, doi: 10.1016/S0140-6736(11)61171-9; Gerald Yonga, "Kenyans Come Together Against Chronic Diseases," *Scientific American* (2014), pp. 20–3; Bo Remenyi et al., "Position Statement of the World Heart Federation on the Prevention and Control of Rheumatic Heart Disease," *Nature Reviews Cardiology* vol. 10 (2013), doi: 10.1038/nrcardio.2013.34.

84. Henry J. Kaiser Family Foundation, "U.S. Global Health Assistance, FY2013 by Program Area."

85. National Research Council, *The U.S. Commitment to Global Health: Recommendations for the New Administration* (Washington, DC: National Academies Press, 2009).

86. John Donnelly, "The President's Emergency Plan for AIDS Relief: How George W. Bush and Aides Came to 'Think Big' on Battling HIV," *Health Affairs* vol. 31 (2012), doi: 10.1377/hlthaff.2012.0408.

87. Tilahun Nigatu, "Integration of HIV and Noncommunicable Diseases in Health Care Delivery in Low- and Middle-Income Countries," *Preventing Chronic Disease* vol. 9 (2012), doi: 10.5888/pcd9.110331.

88. Cesar G. Victora et al., "Maternal and Child Undernutrition: Consequences for Adult Health and Human Capital," *Lancet* vol. 371 (2008), pp. 340–57, doi: 10.1016/S0140-6736(07)61692-4; Matthew Gillman and Janet Rich-Edwards, "The Fetal Origins of Adult Disease: From Skeptic to Convert," *Pediatric and Perinatal Epidemiology* vol. 14 (2000), pp. 192–3.

89. Barbara Janssens et al., "Offering Integrated Care for HIV/AIDS, Diabetes, and Hypertension Within Chronic Disease Clinics in Cambodia," *Bulletin of the World Health Organization* vol. 85 (2007), pp. 880–5, http://www.scielosp.org/pdf/bwho/v85n11/a15v85n11.pdf.

90. Mulindi H. Mwanahamuntu et al., "Advancing Cervical Cancer Prevention Initiatives in Resource-Constrained Settings: Insights From the Cervical Cancer Prevention Program in Zambia," *PLoS Medicine* vol. 8 (2011), doi: 10.1371/journal.pmed.1001032.

91. Miriam Rabkin, Eric Goosby, and Wafaa M. El-Sadr, "Echoing the Lessons of HIV: How to Serve the Millions With Cardiovascular Disease," *Promoting Cardiovascular Health Worldwide* (*Scientific American* special issue, 2014), pp. 30–5.

92. Nigatu, "Integration of HIV and Noncommunicable Diseases in Health Care Delivery in Low- and Middle-Income Countries"; Ed Scholl and Daniel Cothran, "Integrating Family Planning and HIV Services: Programs in Kenya and Ethiopia Lead the Way," AIDSTAR-One Case Study Series (2011), http://www.aidstarone.com/resources/case_study_series/integrating_family_planning_and_hiv_services.

93. Barack Obama, "Millennium Development Goals Summit," speech delivered at United Nations headquarters, New York City, September 2010, http://www.whitehouse.gov/photos-and-video/video/2010/09/22/president-obama-millennium-development-goals-conference.

94. National Intelligence Council, "The Global Infectious Disease Threat and Its Implications for the United States," January 2000, http://fas.org/irp/threat/nie99-17d.htm.

95. White House, "National Security Strategy," May 2010, http://www.whitehouse.gov/sites/default/files/rss_viewer/national_security_strategy.pdf; U.S. Department of State, U.S. Agency for International Development, "Leading Through Civilian Power: The First Quadrennial Diplomacy and Development Review," 2010, http://www.state.gov/documents/organization/153108.pdf; National Intelligence Council, "Strategic Implications of Global Health," December 2008, http://www.state.gov/documents/organization/113592.pdf.

96. Jim Kim, "Why Investing in Poor Countries Helps All of Us," Voices, World Bank, March 24, 2014, http://blogs.worldbank.org/voices/print/why-investing-poor-countries-helps-all-us.

97. Sveinung Fjose, Leo A. Grünfeld, and Chris Green, "SMEs and Growth in Sub-Saharan Africa," MENON Business Economics, June 2010, http://www.norfund.no/getfile.php/Documents/Homepage/Reports%20and%20presentations/Studies%20for%20Norfund/SME%20and%20growth%20MENON%20%5BFINAL%5D.pdf.

98. U.S. International Trade Commission, "Interactive Tariff and Trade DataWeb," http://dataweb.usitc.gov.

99. Tyler Cowen, "What Export-Oriented America Means," American Interest, April 2, 2012, http://www.the-american-interest.com/articles/2012/04/02/what-export-oriented-america-means.

100. Engelgau et al., "Capitalizing on the Demographic Transition"; Stuckler, "Population Causes and Consequences of Leading Chronic Diseases," pp. 273–326.

101. World Economic Forum, "Global Risks 2009: A Global Risk Network Report," January 2009, p. 1, https://members.weforum.org/pdf/globalrisk/2009.pdf.

102. National Research Council, The U.S. Commitment to Global Health: Recommendations for the New Administration.

103. These figures are generated by estimating the burden of death and disability (as measured in DALYs) in 2010 in the forty-nine U.S. priority countries from the cause at issue (i.e, HIV, malaria, or NCDs) and dividing that estimate by U.S. development assistance for health for that cause in the forty-nine countries for the same year. The data sources and methodologies involved are outlined in the Annex to this report, available at www.cfr.org/NCDs_Task_Force.

104. Harley Feldbaum, Kelley Lee, and Joshua Michaud, "Global Health and Foreign Policy," Epidemiologic Reviews vol. 32 (2010), pp. 82–92, doi: 10.1093/epirev/mxq006; U.S. Department of State, "Leading Through Civilian Power."

105. National Intelligence Council, "The Global Infectious Disease Threat and Its Implications for the United States."

106. Henry J. Kaiser Family Foundation, "U.S. Global Health Assistance, FY2013 by Program Area."

107. Ibid.

108. Nikolic, Stanciole, and Zaydman, "Chronic Emergency," p. 9. Lorenzo Rocco et al., "Chronic Diseases and Labor Market Outcomes in Egypt," World Bank Policy Research Working Paper 5575 (2011), doi: 10.1596/1813-9450-5575.

109. Lorenzo Rocco et al., "Chronic Diseases and Labor Market Outcomes in Egypt," World Bank Policy Research Working Paper 5575 (2011), doi: 10.1596/1813-9450-5575.

110. Associated Press, "Middle Class Brazil Family Explains Why They Joined Mass Anti-Government Protests," CBS News, June 27, 2013, http://www.cbsnews.com/news/middle-class-brazil-family-explains-why-they-joined-mass-anti-government-protests; "Chinese Anger Over Pollution Becomes Main Cause of Social Unrest," Bloomberg, March 6, 2013, http://www.bloomberg.com/news/2013-03-06/pollution-passes-land-grievances-as-main-spark-of-china-protests.html.

111. The methodology and data used in this analysis are outlined in the online Annex to this report. The analysis uses a different reference mortality rate, methodology, and date but was inspired by the concept of critical income outlined in Ryan J. Hum et al., "Global Divergence in Critical Income for Adult and Childhood Survival Between 1970 and 2007: An Interpretation of the Preston Curve," *eLife* vol. 1 (2012), doi: 10.7554/eLife.00051.

112. "Teaming Up for Tobacco Control," *Lancet* vol. 372 (2008), p. 345, doi: 10.1016/S0140-6736(08)61133-2.

113. "A Guide in Africa," *Economist*, February 23, 2013, http://www.economist.com/news/business/21572172-why-investors-frontier-markets-need-someone-show-them-around-guide-africa; Josh Kron, "A Middle Class That Is 300 Million Strong," *New York Times,* November 14, 2012, http://www.nytimes.com/2012/11/15/fashion/a-middle-class-that-is-300-million-strong.html.

114. Network of African Science Academies, "Preventing a Tobacco Epidemic in Africa: A Call for Effective Action to Support Health, Social, and Economic Development," National Academies Press, 2014, http://www.nationalacademies.org/asadi/Africa%20Tobacco%20Control-FINAL.pdf.

115. Evan Blecher and Hana Ross, "Tobacco Use in Africa: Tobacco Control Through Prevention," American Cancer Society, 2013, http://global.cancer.org/acs/groups/content/@internationalaffairs/documents/document/acspc-041294.pdf.

116. Adele Baleta, "Africa's Struggle to be Smoke Free," *Lancet* vol. 375 (2010), pp. 107–8, doi: 10.1016/S0140-6736(10)60032-3.

117. United Nations, "Outcome Document: Open Working Group on Sustainable Development Goals," United Nations Working Group for Sustainable Development Goals, July 28, 2014, http://sustainabledevelopment.un.org/focussdgs.html.

118. John W. MacArthur, "Own the Goals: What the Millennium Development Goals Have Accomplished," *Foreign Affairs* vol. 92 (2013), p. 152, http://www.foreignaffairs.com/articles/138821/john-w-mcarthur/own-the-goals; Gorik Ooms et al., "Financing the Millennium Development Goals for Health and Beyond: Sustaining the 'Big Push,'" *Globalization and Health* vol. 6 (2010), p. 17, doi: 10.1186/1744-8603-6-17.

119. Prabhat Jha et al., "Disease Control Priorities in Developing Countries, Third Edition Working Paper #2," Chronic Disease Prevention and Control, Centre for Global Health Research, June 2013, http://www.dcp-3.org/sites/default/files/resources/Chronic%20Disease_Challenge_Final%20Edits_1.pdf.

120. Earl S. Ford et al., "Explaining the Decrease in U.S. Deaths From Coronary Disease, 1980–2000," *New England Journal of Medicine* vol. 356 (2007), doi: 10.1056/NEJMsa053935.

121. Majid Ezzati and Elio Riboli, "Can Noncommunicable Diseases Be Prevented? Lessons From Studies of Populations and Individuals," *Science* vol. 337 (2012), doi: 10.1126/science.1227001.

122. Ibid.

123. Sonia Angell et al., "How Policy Makers Can Advance Cardiovascular Health," *Promoting Cardiovascular Health Worldwide* (*Scientific American* special issue, 2014), pp. 24–9.

124. Christopher P. Howson et al., eds., *Control of Cardiovascular Diseases in Developing Countries: Research, Development, and Institutional Strengthening* (Washington, DC: National Academy Press, 1998).

125. Thomas A. Gaziano and Neha Pagidipati, "Scaling Up Chronic Disease Prevention Interventions in Lower- and Middle-Income Countries," *Annual Review of Public Health* vol. 34 (2013), doi: 10.1146/annurev-publhealth-031912-114402.

126. Simon Stewart and Karen Sliwa, "Preventing CVD in Resource-Poor Areas: Perspectives From the 'Real-World'," *Nature Reviews Cardiology* vol. 6 (2009), pp. 489–92, doi: 10.1038/nrcardio.2009.79.

127. Ibid.

128. Angell et al., "How Policy Makers Can Advance Cardiovascular Health," pp. 24–9; Marc G. Jaffe et al., "Improved Blood Pressure Control Associated With a Large-Scale Hypertension Program," *Journal of American Medical Association* vol. 310 (2013), pp. 699–705, doi: 10.1001/jama.2013.108769.

129. CDC, "The Global Standardized Hypertension Treatment Project," http://www.cdc.gov/globalhealth/ncd/hypertension-treatment.htm.

130. Hans V. Hogerzeil et al., "Promotion of Access to Essential Medicines for Non-Communicable Diseases: Practical Implications of the UN Political Declaration," *Lancet* vol. 381 (2013), pp. 680–9, doi: 10.1016/S0140-6736(12)62128-X.

131. Gaziano and Pagidipati, "Scaling Up Chronic Disease Prevention Interventions in Lower- and Middle-Income Countries," pp. 317–35.

132. Ezzati and Riboli, "Can Noncommunicable Diseases Be Prevented?"

133. Duff Wilson, "Cigarette Giants in Global Fight on Tighter Rules," *New York Times*, November 10, 2010, http://www.nytimes.com/2010/11/14/business/global/14smoke.html.

134. WHO, "Report on the Global Tobacco Epidemic, 2013: Enforcing Bans on Tobacco Advertising, Promotion and Sponsorship," http://apps.who.int/iris/bitstream/10665/85380/1/9789241505871_eng.pdf.

135. Ezzati and Riboli, "Can Noncommunicable Diseases Be Prevented?"

136. Frank A. Sloan and Hellen Gelband, eds., *Cancer Control Opportunities in Low- and Middle-Income Countries* (Washington, DC: National Academies Press, 2007).

137. Fuster and Kelly, eds., *Promoting Cardiovascular Health in the Developing World*, p. 73.

138. Ibid, pp. 103-4.

139. Mattias Öberg et al., "Worldwide Burden of Disease From Exposure to Second-Hand Smoke: A Retrospective Analysis of Data From 192 Countries," *Lancet* vol. 377 (2011), pp. 139–46, doi: 10.1016/S0140-6736(10)61388-8.

140. See Fuster and Kelly, eds., *Promoting Cardiovascular Health in the Developing World*, pp. 320, 338-47, which summarizes the substantial literature that supports the cost-effectiveness of anti-tobacco regulatory interventions, such as taxation, smoke-free public places, restrictions on marketing, and youth cessation.

141. International Agency for Research on Cancer, *IARC Handbooks of Cancer Prevention Tobacco Control, Volume 14: Effectiveness of Tax and Price Policies for Tobacco Control* (Lyon, France: IARC, 2011).

142. World Bank, "Curbing the Epidemic: Governments and the Economics of Tobacco Control," Development in Practice Series, 1999, p. 6; Frank J. Chaloupka et al., "The Taxation of Tobacco Products," in Frank J. Chaloupka and Prabhat Jha, eds., *Tobacco Control in Developing Countries* (Oxford: Oxford University Press, 2000), pp. 2737–72.

143. Omar Shafey et al., "The Tobacco Atlas, Third Edition," American Cancer Society, 2009, p. 82.

144. Evan Blecher, "The Impact of Tobacco Advertising Bans on Consumption in Developing Countries," *Journal of Health Economics* vol. 27 (2008), pp. 930–42.

145. Joanne E. Callinan et al., "Legislative Smoking Bans for Reducing Secondhand Smoke Exposure, Smoking Prevalence and Tobacco Consumption," Cochrane Library (2010), p. 4.

146. "Trends in Current Cigarette Smoking Among High School Students and Adults, United States, 1965–2007," via Centers for Disease Control and Prevention, Smoking & Tobacco Use, http://www.cdc.gov/tobacco/data_statistics/tables/trends/cig_smoking/index.htm.

147. Angell, "How Policy Makers Can Advance Cardiovascular Health," pp. 24–9.

148. "Parties to the WHO Framework Convention on Tobacco Control, March 2014," via WHO Framework Convention on Tobacco Control, http://www.who.int/fctc/signatories_parties/en/index.html.

149. The acronym stands for: Monitor tobacco use and policies; Protect people from secondhand smoke, Offer help to quit; Warn about the dangers of tobacco; Enforce bans on advertising, promotion, and tobacco company sponsorship; and Raise taxes on tobacco products. WHO, "Report on the Global Tobacco Epidemic, 2008: The MPOWER Package," p. 23, http://www.who.int/tobacco/mpower/mpower_report_full_2008.pdf.

150. WHO, "Report on the Global Tobacco Epidemic, 2013: Enforcing Bans on Tobacco Advertising, Promotion and Sponsorship."

151. Bollyky, "Beyond Ratification: The Future of U.S. Engagement on International Tobacco Control."

152. Mohammed K. Ali and Jeffrey P. Koplan, "Promoting Health Through Tobacco Taxation," *Journal of the American Medical Association* vol. 303 (2010).

153. Zinnia B. Dela Peña, "Cigarette, Alcohol Taxes up 81.5%," *Philippine Star*, December 21, 2013, http://www.philstar.com/business/2013/12/21/1270420/cigarette-alcohol-taxes-81.5.

154. Bollyky, "The Tobacco Problem in U.S. Trade"; Editorial Board, "Snuffing Out a Tobacco Exemption in Trans-Pacific Partnership Trade Deal," *Washington Post*, September 17, 2013, http://www.washingtonpost.com/opinions/snuffing-out-a-tobacco-exemption-in-trans-pacific-partnership-trade-deal/2013/09/17/4ed26176-1bf7-11e3-8685-5021e0c41964_story.html.

155. World Bank, "Global Medicines Regulatory Harmonization Discussed," October 18, 2012, http://www.worldbank.org/en/news/feature/2012/10/18/gGlobal-medicines-regulatory-harmonization-discussed.

156. WHO, "Hepatitis B Fact Sheet," 2013, http://www.who.int/mediacentre/factsheets/fs204/en.

157. Logan Brenzel et al., "Chapter 20: Vaccine Preventable Diseases," in *Disease Control Priorities in Developing Countries* (Washington, DC: World Bank, 2006).

158. Sloan and Gelband, eds., *Cancer Control Opportunities in Low- and Middle-Income Countries* (Washington, DC: National Academies Press, 2007).

159. WHO, "Hepatitis B Fact Sheet."

160. Felicia Wu, "Cost-Effectiveness of Interventions to Reduce Aflatoxin Risk" in *Aflatoxins: Finding Solutions for Improved Food Safety*, International Food Policy Research Institute (2013), http://www.ifpri.org/sites/default/files/publications/focus20_11.pdf.

161. WHO, "Hepatitis B Fact Sheet."

162. Ibid; Sandro Vento, "Cancer Control in Africa: Which Priorities?" *Lancet Oncology* vol. 14 (2013), pp. 277–9, doi: 10.1016/S1470-2045(13)70022-6.

163. WHO, "Principles and Considerations for Adding a Vaccine to a National Immunization Program: From Decision to Implementation and Monitoring," 2014, pp. 16, 67, http://apps.who.int/iris/bitstream/10665/111548/1/9789241506892_eng.pdf?ua=1.

164. Brenzel et al., "Chapter 20: Vaccine Preventable Diseases."

165. Ibid.
166. Sloan and Gelband, eds., *Cancer Control in Low-and Middle-Income Countries.*
167. GAVI Alliance, "Human Papillomavirus Vaccine Support: Record Low Price Agreed for HPV Vaccines," 2013, http://www.gavialliance.org/support/nvs/human-papillomavirus-vaccine-support.
168. Ibid.
169. Mark Jit, Marc Brisson, Allison Portnoy, and Raymond Hutubessy, "Cost-effectiveness of Female Human Papillomavirus Vaccination in 179 Countries: A PRIME Modeling Study," *Lancet Global Health* vol. 2 (2014), doi: 10.1016/ S2214-109X(14)70237-2.
170. Seth Berkeley, "Learning From Rwanda," *Project Syndicate*, October 2013, http://www.project-syndicate.org/commentary/seth-berkley-on-how-rwanda-is-beating-cervical-cancer.
171. Tsu et al., "Why the Time is Right to Tackle Breast and Cervical Cancer in Low-Resource Settings."
172. Ibid.
173. Carol E. Levin, Hoang Van Minh, and D. Scott LaMontagne, "Delivery Cost of Human Papillomavirus Vaccination of Young Adolescent Girls in Peru, Uganda and Viet Nam," *Bulletin of the World Health Organization* vol. 91 (2013), pp. 585–92, doi: 10.2471/BLT.12.113837.
174. Jamison et al., "Global Health 2035: A World Converging Within a Generation," pp. 1898–955.
175. Mwanahamuntu et al., "Advancing Cervical Cancer Prevention Initiatives in Resource-Constrained Settings: Insights From the Cervical Cancer Prevention Program in Zambia."
176. Vento, "Cancer Control in Africa: Which Priorities?"
177. Jit et al., "Cost-Effectiveness of Female Human Papillomavirus Vaccination in 179 Countries: A PRIME Modeling Study."
178. Ibid., appendix pp. 17–23, http://download.thelancet.com/mmcs/journals/langlo/ PIIS2214109X14702372/mmc1.pdf?id=haaHNxfqJzEVP55EPWfAu.
179. WHO, "WHO Cervical Cancer Prevention and Control Costing Tool (C4P) User's Guide," 2012, http://www.who.int/immunization/diseases/hpv/C4P_USER_GUIDE_ V1.0.pdf.
180. Jamison et al., "Global Health 2035: A World Converging Within a Generation," pp. 1898–955.
181. Benjamin O. Anderson, "Breast Cancer—Thinking Globally," *Science* vol. 343 (2014), pp. 1403, doi: 10.1126/science.1253344.
182. Sloan and Gelband, eds., *Cancer Control in Low- and Middle-Income Countries.*
183. Ezzati and Riboli, "Can Noncommunicable Diseases Be Prevented?"
184. See Annex, available at www.cfr.org/NCDs_Task_Force.
185. Tsu et al., "Why the Time is Right to Tackle Breast and Cervical Cancer in Low-Resource Settings."
186. Harold Varmus and Harpal S. Kumar, "Addressing the Growing International Challenge of Cancer: A Multinational Perspective," *Science Translational Medicine* vol. 5 (2013), p. 175, doi: 10.1126/scitranslmed.3005899.
187. "Making Cancer Data Count," *Lancet* vol. 383 (2014), p. 1946, doi: 10.1016/ S0140-6736(14)60939-9.
188. Benjamin O. Anderson et al., "Guideline Implementation for Breast Healthcare in Low-Income and Middle-Income Countries: Overview of the Breast Health Global Initiative Global Summit 2007," *Cancer* vol. 113 (2008), pp. 2221–43, doi: 10.1002/ cncr.23844.

189. Tsu et al., "Why the Time is Right to Tackle Breast and Cervical Cancer in Low-Resource Settings."

190. Janssens et al., "Offering Integrated Care for HIV/AIDS, Diabetes and Hypertension Within Chronic Disease Clinics in Cambodia," pp. 880–5.

191. Sabrina Tavernise, "Obesity Studies Tell Two Stories, Both Right," *New York Times*, April 14, 2014, http://www.nytimes.com/2014/04/15/health/obesity-studies-tell-two-stories-both-right.html.

192. Justine E. Leavy, Fiona C. Bull, Michael Rosenberg, and Adrian Bauman, "Physical Activity Mass Media Campaigns and Their Evaluation: A Systematic Review of the Literature 2003–2010," *Health Education Research* vol. 26 (2011), pp. 1060–85, doi: 10.1093/her/cyr069.

193. Khoury et al., "Increasing Homogeneity in Global Food Supplies and the Implications for Food Security," pp. 4001–6.

194. Carl Lachat et al., "Diet and Physical Activity for the Prevention of Noncommunicable Diseases in Low- and Middle-Income Countries: A Systematic Policy Review," *PLoS Med* vol. 10 (2013), doi: 10.1371/journal.pmed.1001465.

195. USAID, "2014 Feed the Future Progress Report: Accelerating Progress to End Global Hunger," May 2014, http://feedthefuture.gov/sites/default/files/resource/files/ftf_progressreport_2014.pdf.

196. Nejmudin Kedir Bilal et al., "Health Extension Workers in Ethiopia: Improved Access and Coverage for the Rural Poor," in P. Chunan-Pole and M. Angwafo, eds, *Yes Africa Can: Success Stories From a Dynamic Continent* (Washington, DC: World Bank, 2011), pp. 433–43.

197. Jha et al., "Disease Control Priorities in Developing Countries, Third Edition Working Paper #2."

198. U.S. Department of Health and Human Services, "Mental Health: A Report of the Surgeon General," 1999.

199. Victoria K. Ngo et al., "Grand Challenges: Integrating Mental Health Care into the Non-Communicable Disease Agenda," *Plos Medicine* vol. 10 (2013), doi: 10.1371/journal.pmed.1001443.

200. Ala Alwan et al., "Global Status Report on Non-Communicable Diseases 2010," WHO, 2011, http://whqlibdoc.who.int/publications/2011/9789240686458_eng.pdf?ua=1.

201. Michael T. Compton, Gail L. Daumit, and Benjamin G. Druss, "Cigarette Smoking and Overweight/Obesity Among Individuals With Serious Mental Illnesses: A Preventive Perspective," *Harvard Review of Psychiatry* vol. 14 (2006).

202. Ngo et al., "Grand Challenges: Integrating Mental Health Care Into the Non-Communicable Disease Agenda."

203. Benjamin G. Druss and Barbara J. Mauer, "Health Care Reform and Care at the Behavioral Health–Primary Care Interface," *Psychiatric Services* vol. 61 (2010), doi: 10.1176/appi.ps.61.11.1087.

204. Charlotte Hanlon et al., "Challenges and Opportunities for Implementing Integrated Mental Health Care: A District Level Situation Analysis from Five Low- and Middle-Income Countries," *PLoS Medicine* vol. 9 (2014), doi: 10.1371/journal.pone.0088437.

205. U.S. Department of State, "U.S.-China Strategic and Economic Dialogue, Outcomes of the Strategic Track," July 12, 2013, http://www.state.gov/r/pa/prs/ps/2013/07/211861.htm; U.S. Department of State, "Joint Statement on Third U.S.-India Strategic Dialogue," June 13, 2012, http://www.state.gov/r/pa/prs/ps/2012/06/192267.htm; U.S. Department of State, "Fourth U.S.-Indonesia Joint Commission Meeting," February 17, 2014, http://www.state.gov/r/pa/prs/ps/2014/02/221714.htm; White House, Office of the Press Secretary, "Fact Sheet: The U.S. Brazil Global Partnership

Dialogue," April 9, 2012, http://www.whitehouse.gov/the-press-office/2012/04/09/fact-sheet-us-brazil-global-partnership-dialogue.

206. Thomas Bollyky and Paul Bollyky, "Obama and the Promotion of International Science," *Science* vol. 338 (2012), doi: 10.1126/science.1230970.

207. Bloom et al., "The Global Economic Burden of Noncommunicable Diseases."

208. Hannah C. Brinsden et al., "Surveys of the Salt Content in UK Bread: Progress Made and Further Reductions Possible," *BMJ Open* vol. 3 (2013), doi: 10.1136/bmjopen-2013-002936.

209. Ibid.

210. Vijay Govindarajan, "A Reverse-Innovation Playbook," *Harvard Business Review*, April 2012, http://hbr.org/2012/04/a-reverse-innovation-playbook/ar/1.

211. Peter Howitt et al., "Technologies for Global Health," *Lancet* vol. 380 (2012), pp. 507–35.

212. WHO "Household Air Pollution and Health: Fact Sheet," March 2014, http://www.who.int/mediacentre/factsheets/fs292/en.

213. Howitt et al., "Technologies for Global Health," pp. 507–35.

214. Ashly D. Black et al., "The Impact of eHealth on the Quality and Safety of Health Care: A Systematic Overview," *PLoS Medicine* vol. 8 (2011), doi: 10.1371/journal.pmed.1000387; Caroline Free et al., "The Effectiveness of Mobile-Health Technologies to Improve Health Care Service Delivery Processes: A Systematic Review and Meta-Analysis," *PLoS Medicine* (2013), doi: 10.1371/journal.pmed.1001363.

215. Hillary Rodham Clinton and Rajiv Shah, "Remarks at USAID Conference on Transforming Development Through Science, Technology and Innovation," U.S. Department of State, July 14, 2010, http://www.state.gov/secretary/20092013clinton/rm/2010/07/144668.htm.

216. USAID, "Grand Challenges for Development," 2014, www.usaid.gov/grandchallenges; USAID, "Development Innovation Ventures," 2014, www.usaid.gov/what-we-do/science-technolog-and-innovation/development-innovation-ventures.

217. Henry J. Kaiser Family Foundation, "Updated: White House Releases FY15 Budget Request," April 22, 2014, http://kff.org/policy-tracker/white-house-releases-fy15-budget-request.

218. Vanessa B. Kerry, Agnes Binagwaho, Jonathan Weigel, and Paul Farmer, "From Aid to Accompaniment: Rules of the Road for Development Assistance," in *The Handbook of Global Health Policy*, eds. Garrett W. Brown, Gaviny Yamey, and Sarah Wamala, (West Sussex: Wiley-Blackwell, 2014); Michael E. Porter, "A Strategy for Health Care Reform—Toward a Value-Based System," *New England Journal of Medicine* 361 (2009): 109-112, 10.1056/NEJMp0904131;Michael E. Porter and Elizabeth Olmsted Teisberg, *Redefining Health Care: Creating Value-Based Competition on Results* (Boston: Harvard Business School Press, 2006).

# Task Force Members

**David B. Agus** is a professor of medicine and engineering at the University of Southern California (USC) Keck School of Medicine and the Viterbi School of Engineering and director of the USC Westside Cancer Center and Center for Applied Molecular Medicine. Agus leads a multidisciplinary team of researchers dedicated to the development and use of technologies to guide doctors in making health-care decisions tailored to individual needs and directs a National Cancer Institute Physical Sciences in Oncology Center at USC. He is a medical oncologist and the cofounder of two personalized medicine companies, Navigenics and Applied Proteomics. Agus is an international leader in new technologies and approaches for personalized health care. His first book, *The End of Illness,* generated international and domestic acclaim following its publication in 2012; it was a number-one *New York Times* and international best seller and the subject of a PBS series of the same name. His most recent publication is *A Short Guide to a Long Life.*

**J. Brian Atwood** is the dean of the Humphrey School of Public Affairs at the University of Minnesota. Atwood served for six years as administrator of the U.S. Agency for International Development (USAID) during the administration of President Bill Clinton. He also led the transition team at the State Department and was undersecretary of state for management prior to his appointment as head of USAID. In 2001, Atwood served on UN Secretary-General Kofi Annan's Panel on Peace Operations. He joined the U.S. Foreign Service in 1966 and served in the American embassies in Ivory Coast and Spain. He served as legislative advisor for foreign and defense policy to Senator Thomas F. Eagleton (D-MO) from 1972 to 1977. During the Carter administration, Atwood served as assistant secretary of state for congressional relations. He was dean of professional studies and academic affairs at the Foreign Service Institute in 1981–82. Atwood was the first president of the National Democratic Institute for International Affairs (NDI) from 1986 to 1993. He received the Secretary of State's Distinguished Service Award in 1999. Atwood's areas of expertise are international development; foreign assistance; the United Nations; UN peacekeeping operations; politics-policy leadership; postconflict reconstruction; and government reform.

**Samuel R. Berger** is chair of Albright Stonebridge Group and is actively involved across the firm's engagements and regions, with a strong focus on Asia, Russia and Central Asia, and the Middle East. Berger has had a distinguished career in both the public and private sectors. From 1997 to 2001, he served as national security adviser to President Bill Clinton, driving policy across a range of issues, including the fight against terrorism; Iraq; advancing the peace process in the Middle East; and strengthening the U.S. relationship with India and China, among others. Previously, he served as deputy national security adviser during President Clinton's first term; as director of national security for the 1992 Clinton-Gore transition; and as senior foreign policy adviser to Governor Clinton during the 1992 presidential campaign. Prior to his service in the Clinton administration, Berger spent sixteen years in the Washington law firm of Hogan & Hartson, where he headed the firm's international group. Berger is an active participant of the U.S. Chamber of Commerce's U.S.-China CEO and Former Senior Officials' Dialogue, the Aspen Strategy Group, and the U.S.-India Strategic Dialogue, and he serves on the international advisory council of the Brookings Doha Center. Berger received his BA from Cornell University and his JD from Harvard Law School.

**Karan Bhatia** joined General Electric Company (GE) as vice president and senior counsel for global government affairs and policy in 2007. In this role, he oversees GE's engagement on public policy issues with governments around the world and works to expand the company's presence in global markets. He previously served in three senior positions in the U.S. government, including deputy U.S. trade representative, assistant secretary of transportation for aviation and international affairs, and deputy undersecretary of commerce for industry and security. Prior to his government service, he was a partner in the Washington, DC, law firm of Wilmer Cutler & Pickering.

**Thomas J. Bollyky** is the senior fellow for global health, economics, and development at the Council on Foreign Relations. He is also an adjunct professor of law at Georgetown University and a consultant for the Bill & Melinda Gates Foundation. Prior to coming to CFR, Bollyky was a fellow at the Center for Global Development and director of intellectual property and innovation at the Office of the U.S. Trade Representative (USTR), where he led the negotiations for parts of the U.S.-Republic of Korea Free Trade Agreement and represented USTR in the negotiations with China on the safety of food and drug imports. He was a Fulbright scholar to South Africa, where he worked as a staff attorney at the AIDS Law Project, and an attorney at Debevoise & Plimpton LLP. Bollyky has testified before the U.S. Senate and his most recent work has appeared in the *New York Times*, *Science*, the *Journal of the American Medical Association*, and *Foreign Affairs*. He serves on the advisory committee for the Clinton Global Initiative. Bollyky received his BA in biology and history at Columbia University and his JD at Stanford Law School. In 2013, the World Economic Forum named Bollyky one of its global leaders under forty.

**Nancy G. Brinker** is regarded as the leader of the global breast cancer movement. Her journey began with a simple promise to her dying sister, Susan G. Komen, that she would do everything possible to end breast cancer forever. In one generation, Susan G. Komen for the Cure has changed the world, investing more than $2.5 billion in breast cancer research, education, screening, and treatment. Brinker's determination to create a world without breast cancer is matched by her passion for enlisting every segment of society—from leaders to citizens—to participate in the battle. In 2009, President Barack Obama honored Brinker with the Presidential Medal of Freedom, the nation's highest civilian honor. Brinker has served as goodwill ambassador for cancer control for the United Nations' World Health Organization, where she continued her mission to ensure cancer control's place at the top of the world health agenda. Brinker has served as U.S. chief of protocol and as U.S. ambassador to Hungary. She is the recipient of numerous awards in recognition of her global work and has been awarded honorary degrees from Duke University, Mount Sinai School of Medicine, Michigan State University, Boston University, and Southern Methodist University. She is a member of the Council on Foreign Relations.

**Binta Niambi Brown** is the executive-in-residence for the New Orleans Startup Fund and PowerMovesNOLA and a Mossavar-Rahmani senior fellow at the Harvard Kennedy School Center for Business and Government. After working for a technology start-up, Brown worked at Cravath, Swaine & Moore. She advised and continues to advise senior management and corporate boards of media, technology, telecom, and entertainment companies. Before leaving to undertake research at Harvard, she was a partner in Kirkland & Ellis and also advised early-stage technology companies. Brown has advised Hillary Clinton, Andrew Cuomo, and members of the Obama administration on a variety of policy matters. She has been recognized as one of the *Root*'s "100 Most Influential African-Americans," *Fortune*'s "40 under 40 business leaders," *Crain's* "New York 40 under 40," and by the World Economic Forum as a Young Global Leader. She has been featured in many publications; is a member of the board of directors of TCI, Inc.; and sits on a handful of advisory and philanthropic boards, including those of 2U Inc., the African Technology Foundation, Human Rights First, the American Theatre Wing, and the New York City Parks Foundation. She is a member of the Council on Foreign Relations and the Clinton Global Initiative.

**Barbara Byrne** is a vice chairman in the investment banking division at Barclays, responsible for leading the firm's global relations with multinational corporate clients. She is a member of Barclays' senior leadership group and is chairman of Barclays' Social Innovation Facility, a cross-business resource dedicated to the development of self-sustaining global commercial solutions to social challenges. Byrne has more than thirty years of financial services experience and has been at the forefront of developing long-standing partnerships with some of Barclays' most important corporate clients. Byrne participates in industry conferences as a forum leader on strategic issues and trends facing the financial sector. She speaks frequently on behalf of women in business, finance, and leadership. She has attended *Fortune*'s Most Powerful Women's Summit for more than ten years and leads Barclays' strategic partnership with the Clinton Global Initiative. In 2012, Byrne was named one of the "100 Women to Watch" by the Cranfield School of Management, and she has gained recognition as one *of American Banker*'s "25 Most Powerful Women in Finance" for the past four years. She is a member of the Council on Foreign Relations and the Women's Forum for the

Economy and Society. She also serves on the New York City board of the British-American Business Council and on the investment committee for the nonprofit organization Catalyst.

**Jean-Paul Chretien** is a U.S. Navy physician who leads the innovation and valuation team in the Division of Integrated Biosurveillance, Armed Forces Health Surveillance Center, in Silver Spring, Maryland. The team develops and assesses novel technologies for tracking health threats to Department of Defense personnel. Previously, he coordinated international partnerships for the DOD's Global Emerging Infectious Surveillance and Response System and served in Helmand province, Afghanistan, from March 2011 to February 2012, leading public health policy and programs for U.S. and NATO forces in the region. Chretien graduated from the U.S. Naval Academy, where he was Truman scholar. He received his MD and PhD in epidemiology, and MHS in biostatistics from the Johns Hopkins University, where he also completed a postdoctoral fellowship in informatics. He trained in preventive medicine at the Walter Reed Army Institute of Research. Chretien's awards include the Rising Star Award from the American College of Preventive Medicine, Best Publication of the Year from the International Society for Disease Surveillance, and the Superior Technology Transfer Award from the U.S. Department of Agriculture.

**Mitchell E. Daniels Jr.** is the twelfth president of Purdue University and the former governor of Indiana. He was elected Indiana's forty-ninth governor in 2004 in his first bid for any elected office, and then was reelected in 2008 with more votes than any candidate for any public office in the state's history. Daniels spearheaded a host of reforms aimed at strengthening the Indiana economy and improving the ethical standards, fiscal condition, and performance of state government. He inherited a budget in deep deficit and left a budget with a large surplus, more than $2 billion in cash reserves, and one of the nation's few AAA state credit ratings. At Purdue, he has prioritized affordability and student success. He froze tuition and committed to maintaining the freeze for at least three years; he called for more accountability and launched the Gallup-Purdue Index, a new method for measuring the value of a college degree; and he invested in a series of initiatives that are expanding Purdue's STEM focus and facilitating the commercialization of faculty discoveries into new businesses and jobs. Previously, Daniels served as

CEO of the Hudson Institute and president of Eli Lilly and Company's North American pharmaceutical operations. He also served as a senior adviser to President Ronald Reagan and as director of the Office of Management and Budget under President George W. Bush.

**Steve Davis**, as president and chief executive officer of PATH, combines his extensive experience as a technology business leader, global health advocate, and social innovator to accelerate great ideas and bring lifesaving solutions to scale. He oversees PATH's work of driving transformative global health innovation to save and improve lives, which reached 219 million people in 2013. Davis's commitment to human rights and global development grew from his early work on refugee programs and policies and from his later focus on Chinese politics and law. He has served as a leader and strategist for a range of private and nonprofit organizations, including as CEO of the global digital media firm Corbis, director of social innovation at McKinsey & Company, and interim CEO of the Infectious Disease Research Institute. Davis is a member of the Council on Foreign Relations and serves on the boards of InterAction and Global Partnerships. He also sits on several advisory groups, including the World Economic Forum's Global Agenda Council on Social Innovation and the Clinton Global Initiative's Global Health Advisory Board. Davis earned his BA from Princeton University, his MA in Chinese studies from the University of Washington, and his JD from Columbia University.

**Thomas E. Donilon** is vice chair of the international law firm O'Melveny & Myers, where he serves on the firm's global governing committee. Donilon is also senior director at the BlackRock Investment Institute. From 2010 to 2013, he served as national security adviser to President Barack Obama. In that capacity, Donilon oversaw the National Security Council staff, chaired the cabinet-level National Security Principals Committee, provided the president's daily national security briefing, and was responsible for the coordination and integration of the U.S. government's foreign policy. He previously served as assistant to the president and principal deputy national security adviser. Donilon is a distinguished fellow at the Council on Foreign Relations, a nonresident senior fellow at the Harvard Kennedy School's Belfer Center for Science and International Affairs, and a member of the U.S. Defense Policy Board and the Central Intelligence Agency's External

Advisory Board. Donilon has worked closely with and advised three U.S. presidents since his first position at the White House in 1977. He has received the Secretary of State's Distinguished Service Award, the National Intelligence Distinguished Public Service Medal, the Department of Defense Medal for Distinguished Public Service, the Chairman of the Joint Chiefs of Staff Joint Distinguished Civilian Service Award, and the CIA's Director's Award.

**Ezekiel J. Emanuel** is the vice provost for global initiatives, the Diane v.S. Levy and Robert M. Levy university professor, and chair of the Department of Medical Ethics and Health Policy at the University of Pennsylvania. He was the founding chair of the Department of Bioethics at the National Institutes of Health and held that position until August 2011. Until January 2011, he served as a special adviser on health policy to the director of the Office of Management and Budget and National Economic Council. He is also a breast oncologist and author. After completing his internship and residency in internal medicine at Boston's Beth Israel Hospital and his oncology fellowship at the Dana-Farber Cancer Institute, he joined the faculty at the Dana-Farber Cancer Institute. Emanuel has published widely on the ethics of clinical research, health-care reform, international research ethics, end-of-life-care issues, euthanasia, the ethics of managed care, and the physician-patient relationship. He is also an op-ed contributor to the *New York Times*. After graduating from Amherst College, he received his MSc from Oxford University in biochemistry. He received his MD from Harvard Medical School and his PhD in political philosophy from Harvard University.

**Daniel R. Glickman** is vice president of the Aspen Institute and executive director of the Aspen Institute Congressional Program. He is co-chair of the Chicago Council on Global Affairs initiative on global food security and a senior fellow at the Bipartisan Policy Center, where he co-chairs the Democracy Project. Prior to joining the Aspen Institute, Glickman served as U.S. secretary of agriculture in the Clinton administration. He also represented the fourth congressional district of Kansas for eighteen years in the U.S. House of Representatives, where he was very involved in federal farm policy on the House Agriculture Committee, served on the House Judiciary Committee, and chaired the House Permanent Select Committee on Intelligence. In addition, Glickman served as chairman of the Motion Picture Association of America, Inc., and director of the Institute of Politics at the Harvard Kennedy School. Glickman has served as president of the Wichita school board; was a partner in the law firm of Sargent, Klenda and Glickman; and worked as a trial attorney at the U.S. Securities and Exchange Commission. He received his bachelor's degree in history from the University of Michigan and his law degree from the George Washington University. He is a member of the Kansas and District of Columbia bars.

**Eric P. Goosby** has dedicated his professional life to fighting HIV/ AIDS, from treating patients to running international programs. After serving for four years in the U.S. State Department as ambassador-at-large and U.S. global AIDS coordinator, overseeing the implementation of the President's Emergency Plan for AIDS Relief (PEPFAR), Goosby returned to the University of California, San Francisco, where he is professor of medicine and director of the Institute for Global Health Delivery and Diplomacy. While at the State Department, he also led the Office of Global Health Diplomacy, advancing the United States' global health mission to improve and save lives and foster sustainability through a shared global responsibility. As chief executive officer and chief medical officer of Pangaea Global AIDS Foundation from 2001 to 2009, he played a key role in the development and implementation of HIV/AIDS national treatment scale-up plans in South Africa, Rwanda, China, and Ukraine. During the Clinton administration, Goosby was director of the Ryan White CARE Act at the U.S. Department of Health and Human Services (HHS), and later he served as deputy director of the White House Office of National AIDS Policy and director of the Office of HIV/AIDS Policy and Infectious Disease Policy at HHS.

**Vanessa Kerry** is the cofounder and CEO of Seed Global Health (Seed), a nonprofit that deploys U.S. health professionals as educators to resource-limited countries to build a pipeline of in-country providers and educators, strengthen health-care capacity, and provide a new type of global diplomacy. She helped establish the Global Health Service Partnership, a public-private partnership among Seed, the Peace Corps, the President's Emergency Plan for AIDS Relief (PEPFAR), and partner countries. For her work, Kerry has been featured in the *Lancet*, *New England Journal of Medicine*, *New York Times*, *Boston Magazine*, and *Medscape*, and on BBC, NPR, and MSNBC. She is a physician at

Massachusetts General Hospital (MGH) and the associate director of partnerships and global initiatives at MGH's Center for Global Health. Academically, Kerry spearheads Harvard Medical School's program in global public policy and social change. She is a Council on Foreign Relations term member and a Draper Richards Kaplan Foundation social entrepreneur. She graduated from Yale University summa cum laude and Harvard Medical School cum laude, completing her internal medicine residency and critical care fellowship at MGH. Kerry earned her master's in health policy, planning, and financing from the London Schools of Economics and of Hygiene and Tropical Medicine.

**Michael J. Klag** is dean of the Johns Hopkins Bloomberg School of Public Health, the oldest and largest independent graduate school of public health in the United States. He served as director of the Division of General Internal Medicine at the Johns Hopkins University School of Medicine and was the first vice dean for clinical investigation there. From 1988 to 2011, he also directed one of the longest-running longitudinal studies in existence, the Precursors Study, which began in 1946. Klag received an honorary doctorate from Juniata College and the James D. Bruce Memorial Award for Distinguished Contributions in Preventive Medicine from the American College of Physicians in 2012. Klag's scientific contributions have been in the prevention and epidemiology of kidney disease, hypertension, and cardiovascular disease. Klag is the author of more than two hundred publications and was the editor in chief of *The Johns Hopkins Family Health Book*. Klag was chair of the NIH Advisory Board on Clinical Research and the Association of Schools and Programs of Public Health. Klag is an internist and epidemiologist who earned his medical degree at the University of Pennsylvania and his MPH degree from the Johns Hopkins School of Hygiene and Public Health

**Risa Lavizzo-Mourey** is president and chief executive officer of the Robert Wood Johnson Foundation, the nation's largest philanthropy dedicated solely to health and health care. A specialist in geriatrics, Lavizzo-Mourey came to the foundation from the University of Pennsylvania, where she served as the Sylvan Eisman professor of medicine and health-care systems. She also directed the University of Pennsylvania's Institute on Aging and was chief of geriatric medicine at the university's School of Medicine. She served as deputy administrator of what is now the Agency for Health Care Research and Quality and worked on the White House Health Care Reform Task Force, co-chairing the working group on quality of care. She also has served on the Task Force on Aging Research, the National Committee for Vital and Health Statistics, and President Bill Clinton's Advisory Commission on Consumer Protection and Quality in the Health Care Industry. Lavizzo-Mourey is a member of the Institute of Medicine of the National Academy of Sciences; the President's Council for Fitness, Sports and Nutrition; and several boards of directors. A graduate of the University of Washington and the State University of New York at Stony Brook, Lavizzo-Mourey received her MD from Harvard Medical School and her MBA from the Wharton School of the University of Pennsylvania.

**Christopher J.L. Murray** is a professor of global health at the University of Washington and institute director of the Institute for Health Metrics and Evaluation (IHME). A physician and health economist, his work has led to the development of a range of new methods and empirical studies to strengthen the basis for population health measurement, measure the performance of public health and medical care systems, and assess the cost effectiveness of health technologies. Murray is a founder of the Global Burden of Disease (GBD) approach, a systematic effort to quantify the comparative magnitude of health loss due to diseases, injuries, and risk factors by age, sex, and geography over time. Prior to IHME, Murray was the executive director of the Evidence and Information for Policy Cluster at the World Health Organization, director of Harvard University's Initiative for Global Health and Center for Population and Development Studies, and the Richard Saltonstall professor of public policy at the Harvard School of Public Health. He holds BA and BSc degrees from Harvard University, a DPhil in international health economics from Oxford University, and an MD from Harvard Medical School.

**Elizabeth G. Nabel** has served as president of the Harvard-affiliated Brigham and Women's Hospital and Brigham and Women's Faulkner Hospital since 2010. A cardiologist and biomedical researcher with more than 250 scientific publications, Nabel is professor of medicine at Harvard Medical School. Nabel brings a unique perspective based on her experience as a physician, research scientist, academic medicine leader, and wellness advocate. This is reflected in Brigham and

Women's strategic plan, which defines a new model of medicine characterized by cross-disciplinary collaboration, patient and family-inclusive care, increased transparency, and innovation in personalized therapies and translational medicine. Prior to joining Brigham and Women's, Nabel served as director of the National Heart, Lung, and Blood Institute. One of Nabel's signature advocacy efforts was the Heart Truth Red Dress campaign, which raises heart awareness in women. Nabel attended Cornell Medical College and completed her cardiovascular training at Brigham and Women's Hospital.

**David Satcher** is director of the Satcher Health Leadership Institute, which was established in 2006 at the Morehouse School of Medicine in Atlanta, Georgia. Satcher was sworn in as the sixteenth surgeon general of the United States in 1998 and served until 2002. He also served as the tenth assistant secretary for health in the Department of Health and Human Services, making him only the second person in history to have held both positions simultaneously. His tenure of public service also includes serving as director of the Centers for Disease Control and Prevention (CDC). He was the first person to have served as director of the CDC and then surgeon general of the United States. Satcher has held top leadership positions at the Charles R. Drew University for Medicine and Science, Meharry Medical College, and the Morehouse School of Medicine.

**Donna E. Shalala** is president and professor of political science at the University of Miami. One of the country's first Peace Corps volunteers, she served in Iran from 1962 to 1964. She has held tenured professorships at Columbia University, the City University of New York (CUNY), and the University of Wisconsin–Madison. She served as president of Hunter College of the City University of New York from 1980 to 1987 and as chancellor of the University of Wisconsin–Madison from 1987 to 1993. In 1993, President Bill Clinton appointed her U.S. secretary of health and human services (HHS), which she served as for eight years, becoming the longest-serving HHS secretary in U.S. history. She is the recipient of more than four dozen honorary degrees and a host of other honors, including the Presidential Medal of Freedom in 2008 and the Nelson Mandela Award for Health and Human Rights in 2010. Shalala is a member of the Council on Foreign Relations and has been elected to the American Academy of Arts and Sciences, the

American Philosophical Society, and the Institute of Medicine of the
National Academy of Sciences. She received her AB degree from Western College for Women and earned her PhD from the Maxwell School
of Citizenship and Public Affairs at Syracuse University.

**Ira S. Shapiro** is the president of Ira Shapiro Global Strategies LLC,
a consulting firm focused on international trade law and policy issues,
with a principal focus on U.S.-Japan relations. He is also chairman of the
National Association of Japan-America Societies. Shapiro previously
served in the Clinton administration as general counsel to the Office
of the U.S. Trade Representative, where he played an important role in
completing the North American Free Trade Agreement and the multilateral Uruguay Round. He then served as chief U.S. trade negotiator
to Japan and Canada, with ambassadorial rank, and he was also heavily involved in the successful negotiation of the Framework Convention
on Tobacco Control, the first global health treaty negotiated under the
auspices of the World Health Organization. He is the author of an influential article contending that tobacco products should be treated as an
exception to the normal trade rules because of their lethal nature. Prior
to serving in the Clinton administration, Shapiro held senior staff positions in the U.S. Senate for twelve years. Shapiro received his BA from
Brandeis University; his MA in political science from the University of
California, Berkeley; and his JD from the University of Pennsylvania
Law School.

**Tommy G. Thompson** is a former secretary of the U.S. Department
of Health and Human Services (HHS), serving from 2001 to 2005, and
a four-term governor of Wisconsin, serving from 1987 to 2001. From
2005 to 2009, Thompson served as a senior adviser at the consulting
firm Deloitte and Touche USA LLP, and he was the founding independent chairman of the Deloitte Center for Health Solutions. Thompson
previously served as a senior partner at Akin, Gump, Strauss, Hauer,
& Feld LLP from 2005 to 2012; as chairman of the board of directors
of Logistics Health, Inc., from January 2011 to May 2011; and as the
company's president from February 2005 to January 2011. He currently
serves on the board of directors of CareView Communications, Inc.;
Centene Corporation; C.R. Bard, Inc.; United Therapeutics Corporation; Cytori Therapeutics, Inc.; and TherapeuticsMD, Inc. Thompson has received numerous awards for his public service, including the

Anti-Defamation League's Distinguished Public Service Award, the Friend of Zion Award, *Governing*'s Public Official of the Year Award, and the Horatio Alger Award. Thompson has also served as chairman of the National Governors' Association, the Education Commission of the States, and the Midwestern Governors' Conference. Thompson received his BSs and JD from the University of Wisconsin, Madison.

# Task Force Observers

**Yanzhong Huang** is senior fellow for global health at the Council on Foreign Relations and an associate professor and director of the Center for Global Health Studies at the Seton Hall University School of Diplomacy and International Relations. Huang is the founding editor of *Global Health Governance: The Scholarly Journal for the New Health Security Paradigm*. He has written extensively on global health governance, health diplomacy and health security, and public health in China. He has published numerous reports, journal articles, and book chapters, including articles in *Survival*, *Foreign Affairs*, and *Bioterrorism and Biosecurity*, as well as op-ed pieces in the *New York Times*, *International Herald Tribune*, and the *Lancet*, among others. He is author of *Governing Health in Contemporary China*. He is frequently consulted by major media outlets, the private sector, and governmental and nongovernmental organizations on global health issues and China. In March 2012, he was listed by *InsideJersey* as one of New Jersey's "20 Exceptional Intellectuals Who Are Changing the World." Huang has taught at Barnard College and Columbia University. He received his BA and MA degrees from Fudan University and his PhD degree from the University of Chicago.

**Laura Solia** is a public health professional committed to using the power of partnerships to advance solutions to global challenges. She spent the last five years at the Clinton Global Initiative (CGI), where she served as the head of CGI's Global Health Track. In this role, Solia was responsible for the strategic development of CGI's global health agenda and year-round programming. She worked with a wide array of NGOs, foundations, private companies, and governments to facilitate the development of innovative partnerships and "Commitments to Action" addressing critical global health issues, and chaired CGI's Noncommunicable Diseases Action Network. Solia began her career working with grassroots nonprofits in Central America and Africa, focused on community development, nutrition, and public health. She holds a BA in politics and public health policy from New York University (NYU) and an MSc in global affairs from NYU's Center for Global Affairs.

# Independent Task Force Reports

*Published by the Council on Foreign Relations*

*North America: Time for a New Focus*
David H. Petraeus and Robert B. Zoellick, Chairs; Shannon K. O'Neil, Project Director
Independent Task Force No. 71 (2014)

*Defending an Open, Global, Secure, and Resilient Internet*
John D. Negroponte and Samuel J. Palmisano, Chairs; Adam Segal, Project Director
Independent Task Force Report No. 70 (2013)

*U.S.-Turkey Relations: A New Partnership*
Madeleine K. Albright and Stephen J. Hadley, Chairs; Steven A. Cook, Project Director
Independent Task Force Report No. 69 (2012)

*U.S. Education Reform and National Security*
Joel I. Klein and Condoleezza Rice, Chairs; Julia Levy, Project Director
Independent Task Force Report No. 68 (2012)

*U.S. Trade and Investment Policy*
Andrew H. Card and Thomas A. Daschle, Chairs; Edward Alden and Matthew J. Slaughter,
Project Directors
Independent Task Force Report No. 67 (2011)

*Global Brazil and U.S.-Brazil Relations*
Samuel W. Bodman and James D. Wolfensohn, Chairs; Julia E. Sweig, Project Director
Independent Task Force Report No. 66 (2011)

*U.S. Strategy for Pakistan and Afghanistan*
Richard L. Armitage and Samuel R. Berger, Chairs; Daniel S. Markey, Project Director
Independent Task Force Report No. 65 (2010)

*U.S. Policy Toward the Korean Peninsula*
Charles L. Pritchard and John H. Tilelli Jr., Chairs; Scott A. Snyder, Project Director
Independent Task Force Report No. 64 (2010)

*U.S. Immigration Policy*
Jeb Bush and Thomas F. McLarty III, Chairs; Edward Alden, Project Director
Independent Task Force Report No. 63 (2009)

*U.S. Nuclear Weapons Policy*
William J. Perry and Brent Scowcroft, Chairs; Charles D. Ferguson, Project Director
Independent Task Force Report No. 62 (2009)

*Confronting Climate Change: A Strategy for U.S. Foreign Policy*
George E. Pataki and Thomas J. Vilsack, Chairs; Michael A. Levi, Project Director
Independent Task Force Report No. 61 (2008)

*U.S.-Latin America Relations: A New Direction for a New Reality*
Charlene Barshefsky and James T. Hill, Chairs; Shannon O'Neil, Project Director
Independent Task Force Report No. 60 (2008)

*U.S.-China Relations: An Affirmative Agenda, A Responsible Course*
Carla A. Hills and Dennis C. Blair, Chairs; Frank Sampson Jannuzi, Project Director
Independent Task Force Report No. 59 (2007)

*National Security Consequences of U.S. Oil Dependency*
John Deutch and James R. Schlesinger, Chairs; David G. Victor, Project Director
Independent Task Force Report No. 58 (2006)

*Russia's Wrong Direction: What the United States Can and Should Do*
John Edwards and Jack Kemp, Chairs; Stephen Sestanovich, Project Director
Independent Task Force Report No. 57 (2006)

*More than Humanitarianism: A Strategic U.S. Approach Toward Africa*
Anthony Lake and Christine Todd Whitman, Chairs; Princeton N. Lyman and J. Stephen
Morrison, Project Directors
Independent Task Force Report No. 56 (2006)

*In the Wake of War: Improving Post-Conflict Capabilities*
Samuel R. Berger and Brent Scowcroft, Chairs; William L. Nash, Project Director; Mona K.
Sutphen, Deputy Director
Independent Task Force Report No. 55 (2005)

*In Support of Arab Democracy: Why and How*
Madeleine K. Albright and Vin Weber, Chairs; Steven A. Cook, Project Director
Independent Task Force Report No. 54 (2005)

*Building a North American Community*
John P. Manley, Pedro Aspe, and William F. Weld, Chairs; Thomas d'Aquino, Andrés
Rozental, and Robert Pastor, Vice Chairs; Chappell H. Lawson, Project Director
Independent Task Force Report No. 53 (2005)

*Iran: Time for a New Approach*
Zbigniew Brzezinski and Robert M. Gates, Chairs; Suzanne Maloney, Project Director
Independent Task Force Report No. 52 (2004)

*An Update on the Global Campaign Against Terrorist Financing*
Maurice R. Greenberg, Chair; William F. Wechsler and Lee S. Wolosky, Project Directors
Independent Task Force Report No. 40B (Web-only release, 2004)

*Renewing the Atlantic Partnership*
Henry A. Kissinger and Lawrence H. Summers, Chairs; Charles A. Kupchan, Project Director
Independent Task Force Report No. 51 (2004)

*Iraq: One Year After*
Thomas R. Pickering and James R. Schlesinger, Chairs; Eric P. Schwartz, Project Consultant
Independent Task Force Report No. 43C (Web-only release, 2004)

*Nonlethal Weapons and Capabilities*
Paul X. Kelley and Graham Allison, Chairs; Richard L. Garwin, Project Director
Independent Task Force Report No. 50 (2004)

*New Priorities in South Asia: U.S. Policy Toward India, Pakistan, and Afghanistan (Chairmen's Report)*
Marshall Bouton, Nicholas Platt, and Frank G. Wisner, Chairs; Dennis Kux and Mahnaz Ispahani, Project Directors
Independent Task Force Report No. 49 (2003)
Cosponsored with the Asia Society

*Finding America's Voice: A Strategy for Reinvigorating U.S. Public Diplomacy*
Peter G. Peterson, Chair; Kathy Bloomgarden, Henry Grunwald, David E. Morey, and Shibley Telhami, Working Committee Chairs; Jennifer Sieg, Project Director; Sharon Herbstman, Project Coordinator
Independent Task Force Report No. 48 (2003)

*Emergency Responders: Drastically Underfunded, Dangerously Unprepared*
Warren B. Rudman, Chair; Richard A. Clarke, Senior Adviser; Jamie F. Metzl, Project Director
Independent Task Force Report No. 47 (2003)

*Iraq: The Day After (Chairs' Update)*
Thomas R. Pickering and James R. Schlesinger, Chairs; Eric P. Schwartz, Project Director
Independent Task Force Report No. 43B (Web-only release, 2003)

*Burma: Time for Change*
Mathea Falco, Chair
Independent Task Force Report No. 46 (2003)

*Afghanistan: Are We Losing the Peace?*
Marshall Bouton, Nicholas Platt, and Frank G. Wisner, Chairs; Dennis Kux and Mahnaz Ispahani, Project Directors
Chairman's Report of an Independent Task Force (2003)
Cosponsored with the Asia Society

*Meeting the North Korean Nuclear Challenge*
Morton I. Abramowitz and James T. Laney, Chairs; Eric Heginbotham, Project Director
Independent Task Force Report No. 45 (2003)

*Chinese Military Power*
Harold Brown, Chair; Joseph W. Prueher, Vice Chair; Adam Segal, Project Director
Independent Task Force Report No. 44 (2003)

*Iraq: The Day After*
Thomas R. Pickering and James R. Schlesinger, Chairs; Eric P. Schwartz, Project Director
Independent Task Force Report No. 43 (2003)

*Threats to Democracy: Prevention and Response*
Madeleine K. Albright and Bronislaw Geremek, Chairs; Morton H. Halperin, Director;
Elizabeth Frawley Bagley, Associate Director
Independent Task Force Report No. 42 (2002)

*America—Still Unprepared, Still in Danger*
Gary Hart and Warren B. Rudman, Chairs; Stephen E. Flynn, Project Director
Independent Task Force Report No. 41 (2002)

*Terrorist Financing*
Maurice R. Greenberg, Chair; William F. Wechsler and Lee S. Wolosky, Project Directors
Independent Task Force Report No. 40 (2002)

*Enhancing U.S. Leadership at the United Nations*
David Dreier and Lee H. Hamilton, Chairs; Lee Feinstein and Adrian Karatnycky, Project
Directors
Independent Task Force Report No. 39 (2002)
Cosponsored with Freedom House

*Improving the U.S. Public Diplomacy Campaign in the War Against Terrorism*
Carla A. Hills and Richard C. Holbrooke, Chairs; Charles G. Boyd, Project Director
Independent Task Force Report No. 38 (Web-only release, 2001)

*Building Support for More Open Trade*
Kenneth M. Duberstein and Robert E. Rubin, Chairs; Timothy F. Geithner, Project Director;
Daniel R. Lucich, Deputy Project Director
Independent Task Force Report No. 37 (2001)

*Beginning the Journey: China, the United States, and the WTO*
Robert D. Hormats, Chair; Elizabeth Economy and Kevin Nealer, Project Directors
Independent Task Force Report No. 36 (2001)

*Strategic Energy Policy Update*
Edward L. Morse, Chair; Amy Myers Jaffe, Project Director
Independent Task Force Report No. 33B (2001)
Cosponsored with the James A. Baker III Institute for Public Policy of Rice University

*Testing North Korea: The Next Stage in U.S. and ROK Policy*
Morton I. Abramowitz and James T. Laney, Chairs; Robert A. Manning, Project Director
Independent Task Force Report No. 35 (2001)

*The United States and Southeast Asia: A Policy Agenda for the New Administration*
J. Robert Kerrey, Chair; Robert A. Manning, Project Director
Independent Task Force Report No. 34 (2001)

*Strategic Energy Policy: Challenges for the 21st Century*
Edward L. Morse, Chair; Amy Myers Jaffe, Project Director
Independent Task Force Report No. 33 (2001)
Cosponsored with the James A. Baker III Institute for Public Policy of Rice University

*A Letter to the President and a Memorandum on U.S. Policy Toward Brazil*
Stephen Robert, Chair; Kenneth Maxwell, Project Director
Independent Task Force Report No. 32 (2001)

*State Department Reform*
Frank C. Carlucci, Chair; Ian J. Brzezinski, Project Coordinator
Independent Task Force Report No. 31 (2001)
Cosponsored with the Center for Strategic and International Studies

*U.S.-Cuban Relations in the 21st Century: A Follow-on Report*
Bernard W. Aronson and William D. Rogers, Chairs; Julia Sweig and Walter Mead, Project
Directors
Independent Task Force Report No. 30 (2000)

*Toward Greater Peace and Security in Colombia: Forging a Constructive U.S. Policy*
Bob Graham and Brent Scowcroft, Chairs; Michael Shifter, Project Director
Independent Task Force Report No. 29 (2000)
Cosponsored with the Inter-American Dialogue

*Future Directions for U.S. Economic Policy Toward Japan*
Laura D'Andrea Tyson, Chair; M. Diana Helweg Newton, Project Director
Independent Task Force Report No. 28 (2000)

*First Steps Toward a Constructive U.S. Policy in Colombia*
Bob Graham and Brent Scowcroft, Chairs; Michael Shifter, Project Director
Interim Report (2000)
Cosponsored with the Inter-American Dialogue

*Promoting Sustainable Economies in the Balkans*
Steven Rattner, Chair; Michael B.G. Froman, Project Director
Independent Task Force Report No. 27 (2000)

*Non-Lethal Technologies: Progress and Prospects*
Richard L. Garwin, Chair; W. Montague Winfield, Project Director
Independent Task Force Report No. 26 (1999)

*Safeguarding Prosperity in a Global Financial System:*
*The Future International Financial Architecture*
Carla A. Hills and Peter G. Peterson, Chairs; Morris Goldstein, Project Director
Independent Task Force Report No. 25 (1999)
Cosponsored with the International Institute for Economics

*U.S. Policy Toward North Korea: Next Steps*
Morton I. Abramowitz and James T. Laney, Chairs; Michael J. Green, Project Director
Independent Task Force Report No. 24 (1999)

*Reconstructing the Balkans*
Morton I. Abramowitz and Albert Fishlow, Chairs; Charles A. Kupchan, Project Director
Independent Task Force Report No. 23 (Web-only release, 1999)

*Strengthening Palestinian Public Institutions*
Michel Rocard, Chair; Henry Siegman, Project Director; Yezid Sayigh and Khalil Shikaki,
Principal Authors
Independent Task Force Report No. 22 (1999)

*U.S. Policy Toward Northeastern Europe*
Zbigniew Brzezinski, Chair; F. Stephen Larrabee, Project Director
Independent Task Force Report No. 21 (1999)

*The Future of Transatlantic Relations*
Robert D. Blackwill, Chair and Project Director
Independent Task Force Report No. 20 (1999)

*U.S.-Cuban Relations in the 21st Century*
Bernard W. Aronson and William D. Rogers, Chairs; Walter Russell Mead, Project Director
Independent Task Force Report No. 19 (1999)

*After the Tests: U.S. Policy Toward India and Pakistan*
Richard N. Haass and Morton H. Halperin, Chairs
Independent Task Force Report No. 18 (1998)
Cosponsored with the Brookings Institution

*Managing Change on the Korean Peninsula*
Morton I. Abramowitz and James T. Laney, Chairs; Michael J. Green, Project Director
Independent Task Force Report No. 17 (1998)

*Promoting U.S. Economic Relations with Africa*
Peggy Dulany and Frank Savage, Chairs; Salih Booker, Project Director
Independent Task Force Report No. 16 (1998)

*U.S. Middle East Policy and the Peace Process*
Henry Siegman, Project Coordinator
Independent Task Force Report No. 15 (1997)

*Differentiated Containment: U.S. Policy Toward Iran and Iraq*
Zbigniew Brzezinski and Brent Scowcroft, Chairs; Richard W. Murphy, Project Director
Independent Task Force Report No. 14 (1997)

*Russia, Its Neighbors, and an Enlarging NATO*
Richard G. Lugar, Chair; Victoria Nuland, Project Director
Independent Task Force Report No. 13 (1997)

*Rethinking International Drug Control: New Directions for U.S. Policy*
Mathea Falco, Chair
Independent Task Force Report No. 12 (1997)

*Financing America's Leadership: Protecting American Interests and Promoting American Values*
Mickey Edwards and Stephen J. Solarz, Chairs; Morton H. Halperin, Lawrence J. Korb,
and Richard M. Moose, Project Directors
Independent Task Force Report No. 11 (1997)
Cosponsored with the Brookings Institution